Indirect Questioning in Sample Surveys

Arijit Chaudhuri • Tasos C. Christofides

Indirect Questioning in Sample Surveys

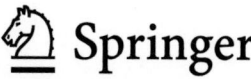

Arijit Chaudhuri
Applied Statistics Unit
Indian Statistical Institute
Kolkata, India

Tasos C. Christofides
Department of Mathematics and Statistics
University of Cyprus
Nicosia, Cyprus

ISBN 978-3-642-36275-0   ISBN 978-3-642-36276-7 (eBook)
DOI 10.1007/978-3-642-36276-7
Springer Heidelberg New York Dordrecht London

Library of Congress Control Number: 2013946203

Mathematics Subject Classification (2010): 62D05, 62P25

© Springer-Verlag Berlin Heidelberg 2013
This work is subject to copyright. All rights are reserved by the Publisher, whether the whole or part of the material is concerned, specifically the rights of translation, reprinting, reuse of illustrations, recitation, broadcasting, reproduction on microfilms or in any other physical way, and transmission or information storage and retrieval, electronic adaptation, computer software, or by similar or dissimilar methodology now known or hereafter developed. Exempted from this legal reservation are brief excerpts in connection with reviews or scholarly analysis or material supplied specifically for the purpose of being entered and executed on a computer system, for exclusive use by the purchaser of the work. Duplication of this publication or parts thereof is permitted only under the provisions of the Copyright Law of the Publisher's location, in its current version, and permission for use must always be obtained from Springer. Permissions for use may be obtained through RightsLink at the Copyright Clearance Center. Violations are liable to prosecution under the respective Copyright Law.
The use of general descriptive names, registered names, trademarks, service marks, etc. in this publication does not imply, even in the absence of a specific statement, that such names are exempt from the relevant protective laws and regulations and therefore free for general use.
While the advice and information in this book are believed to be true and accurate at the date of publication, neither the authors nor the editors nor the publisher can accept any legal responsibility for any errors or omissions that may be made. The publisher makes no warranty, express or implied, with respect to the material contained herein.

Printed on acid-free paper

Springer is part of Springer Science+Business Media (www.springer.com)

To Bulu
　AC

To Liana, Andrea, Christoforos
　TCC

Preface

Asking questions about sensitive and stigmatizing characteristics in surveys of human populations is not an easy matter. Gathering information on issues like sexual orientation, drunkenness, HIV positivity, experience in induced abortion, maltreatment of spouse, habits of wilful tax evasion, bribery, cheating, and fraud by means of direct questions and conventional survey methodology is likely to produce large nonsampling errors particularly due to nonresponse. People are not willing to provide information which might be considered as incriminating and stigmatizing. In cases they agreed to participate in such a survey, it is very reasonable to assume that many of them give false answers and provide misleading information.

Warner (1965) was the first to offer a way out as a pioneer with his Randomized Response Technique. A participant in a survey employing his technique, using a so-called randomization device, provides information from which it is not possible to infer whether he/she has the stigmatizing characteristic and thus his/her privacy is protected. However, based on the information collected from all participants, it is possible to make inferences about the prevalence of the stigmatizing attribute. This principle, namely that the information provided by a participant is not adequate to make inferences about his/her status as related to the sensitive characteristic but the information collected from all participants together is sufficient to estimate certain parameters of the population, is the one which governs all indirect questioning techniques devised so far.

Prospective readers may be familiar with the three treatises, namely (1) Randomized Response and Indirect Questioning Techniques in Surveys (Chapman & Hall, CRC Press, Boca Raton, Florida, USA, 2011) by Arijit Chaudhuri, (2) Randomized Response: Theory and Techniques (Marcel Dekker, NY. USA, 1988) by Arijit Chaudhuri and Rahul Mukerjee, and (3) Randomized Response: A method for Sensitive Surveys (Sage, London, 1986) by J.A.Fox and P.E.Tracy.

Warner and most of his followers did not clarify if their theories are related to a theoretical or a survey population of labeled individuals. Consequently most of the published works including (2) and (3) above dealt with analysis confined to simple random sampling with replacement alone. A few published papers and Chap. 7 in Chaudhuri and Mukerjee (1988) considered labeled finite survey populations and general sampling schemes allowing selection without replacement and even selection with unequal or varying probabilities. The monograph (1) noted above provides a comprehensive review opening an avenue for further research in theory and practice in randomized response. It is a research publication out and out. Its emphasis is on thrashing out the point that for every randomized response technique employed in respect of the people selected in a sample, no matter how, data analysis is possible to throw up unbiased estimators for the proportion of people bearing a sensitive attribute in a community throwing up estimated measures of accuracy in estimation only provided that every person is given a positive inclusion-probability in a sample and that every pair of distinct persons also has a positive inclusion-probability in a sample. Chaudhuri (2011) and Chaudhuri and Mukerjee (1988) covered estimation of survey population totals of stigmatizing variables. In addition, taking account of certain emerging criticisms of randomized response techniques in general, alternative data-gathering procedures in indirect manners are also briefly studied by Chaudhuri's (2011) text.

However, recognizing that the monographs above involve a good deal of analytical sophistication not quite tasteful to social scientists enjoying less pleasure in their perusal but really more interested in the essentials of these Indirect Techniques for gathering sensitive data, the present monograph attempts at presenting a compendium of useful techniques with straightforward analytical tools in rather condensed forms. Although randomized response techniques account for the lion's share of indirect questioning, more recent approaches move away from the idea of using a randomization device. This monograph attempts to give the most basic and important aspects of indirect questioning. In addition to randomized response and other indirect questioning approaches such as the item count technique, the nominative technique, and the three-card method which have been known for quite some time, this monograph contains modern approaches such as non-randomized techniques and surveys with negative questions not to be found in any of the three monographs mentioned above.

In this book, the issue of the protection of privacy has a prominent place. But here we just do not view it as a concept on which one builds mathematical formulas and numerical indicators. We put emphasis on the perceived protection of privacy, i.e., the protection of privacy as how participants perceive it. Although the book does not offer any solutions to the issue of quantification of the perceived protection of privacy, we firmly believe that it will provide incentives to researchers, in particular social scientists to join forces with mathematical statisticians on this important issue.

Kolkata, India Arijit Chaudhuri
Nicosia, Cyprus Tasos C. Christofides
July 2013

Acknowledgments

I am indebted to the Director, Indian Statistical Institute and my colleagues in Applied Statistics Unit for offering me certain requisite spare time to complete writing this monograph.

Arijit Chaudhuri

I am indebted to the University of Cyprus for creating the academic environment that allows faculty members to author manuscripts such as this one.

Tasos C. Christofides

Contents

1 **A Plea for Indirect Questioning: Stigmatizing Issues of Social Relevance** 1
   1.1 Introduction 1
   1.2 Real and Hypothetical Examples to Justify the Need for Indirect Methods 3
   References 5

2 **Specification of Qualitative and Quantitative Parameters Demanding Estimation** 9
   2.1 Introduction 9
   2.2 Estimating Parameters 16
   2.3 How to Sample? 19
   2.4 How to Gather Sensitive Data? 19
   References 19

3 **Various Indirect Questioning Techniques** 21
   3.1 Introduction 21
   3.2 Randomized Response Technique: Its Rationale 22
   3.3 Item Count Technique: Its Rationale 24
   3.4 Nominative Technique: Its Rationale 24
   3.5 The Three Card Method: Its Rationale 25
   3.6 Non Randomized Models 25
   3.7 Surveys with Negative Questions 26
   References 26

4 **Randomized Response Techniques to Capture Qualitative Features** 29
   4.1 Introduction 29
   4.2 Warner's, Simmons's, Kuk's, Forced Response, and Christofides's RRT 31
   4.3 Related Estimation in SRSWR and Sophisticated Sampling 34

4.4	Certain Alternative RR Procedures with Rationales	53
	4.4.1 Dalenius and Vitale (1974) Approach	53
	4.4.2 Liu, Chow, and Mosley's (1975) RR Device	57
	4.4.3 Mangat and Singh's (1990) RR Device	59
	4.4.4 Mangat's (1992) RR Device as Modified by Chaudhuri (2011)	61
	4.4.5 Mangat, Singh, and Singh's (1992) Device	62
	4.4.6 Mangat's (1994) Device	63
	4.4.7 Singh and Joarder's (1997a) RR Device	64
	4.4.8 Randomized Response Using the Poisson Distribution	65
4.5	Alternative Randomized Response Generation	69
4.6	Estimation for more than one Sensitive Characteristics	77
	4.6.1 Estimating Two Characteristics	78
	4.6.2 The Crossed Model	81
	4.6.3 Multiple Characteristics	83
4.7	Some Aspects of Bayesian Approach in Analyzing RR Data	86
4.8	Further Developments on Randomized Response	90
References		91

5 Quantitative Issues Bearing Stigma: Parameter Estimation — 95

5.1	Introduction	95
5.2	Theory of Estimating Totals/Means of Stigmatizing Characteristics	96
	5.2.1 Device I	97
	5.2.2 Device II	99
5.3	Optional Randomized Response	103
	5.3.1 The Approach of Huang (2010)	105
	5.3.2 The Approach of Gupta, Shabbir and Sehra (2010)	107
	5.3.3 Optional Randomized Response for Complex Sampling Designs	109
References		112

6 Indirect Techniques as Alternatives to Randomized Response — 115

6.1	Introduction	115
6.2	The Item Count Technique	117
	6.2.1 Revised Version of the Item Count Technique	117
	6.2.2 Three Sample Item Count Technique	123
	6.2.3 Item Count Technique for Quantitative Sensitive Characteristics	127
6.3	The Nominative Technique	129
6.4	The Three-Card Method	132
6.5	Non Randomized Models	134
6.6	Surveys with Negative Questions	144
References		147

7	**Protection of Privacy**		151
	7.1 Introduction		151
	7.2 Measures of Jeopardy		152
	7.3 Protection of Privacy in Case of Quantitative Sensitive Characteristics		162
		7.3.1 Randomized Device I	164
		7.3.2 Randomized Response Device II	166
	7.4 Perceived Protection of Privacy		167
	References		170

Index 173

Chapter 1
A Plea for Indirect Questioning: Stigmatizing Issues of Social Relevance

Abstract Collecting data on human populations by means of sample surveys is not an easy task. Survey practitioners often experience difficulties in collecting reliable data due to various sources of nonsampling error and in particular due to nonresponse. In case the issues under investigation are of sensitive nature, such as issues on sexual orientation, tax evasion, or involvement in criminal activities, people are reluctant to participate, and even if they agree to participate, false or misleading answers are given by many of them. Indirect questioning techniques offer a solution to this problem. These are techniques designed in such a way that the information provided by a participant is not incriminating and thus his/her privacy is protected. However, based on the information collected from all participants, the investigator is able to estimate parameters of interest related to the sensitive characteristic. In this chapter we make a case in favor of the use of indirect questioning techniques. We briefly discuss hypothetical as well as real examples where the methodology presented in this book can be implemented.

1.1 Introduction

With time advancing, human civilization is rapidly progressing. Keeping pace with it, many social taboos are quickly disappearing. Yet, the society seems not to be permissive enough. Many practices are still found not to capture social approbation. For example, social scientists deem it discourteous to ask a stranger chosen in a sample if he/she is a habitual gambler or a tax evader or an exorbitantly drunken driver of a motor vehicle or engaged in any one or more similar illegal and/or unethical practices. Overcoming the delicacy, even if one plucks enough courage to put up a brave face to enquire about such traits in a chosen respondent, honest answers are frequently in short supply. People fight shy and either refuse to answer, or the responses often are suspected to be far from the truth in their revelations. Warner (1965) first published a technique of indirect questioning. This inaugurated an era of fruitful coverage of data on sensitive items in meaningful studies. In addition to asking questions of sensitive nature, nowadays the issue of personal data protection makes it necessary to employ techniques which guarantee that no would be in a position to make inferences about the status or personal data of an individual, even if the status in question is not stigmatizing at all.

Our purpose is to develop a handbook of procedures to estimate parameters relating to items bearing social stigmas for human subjects. It is intended to be a compendium on how to gather sensitive information in sample surveys from persons by asking indirect questions or by employing certain techniques that essentially mask one's answer. The use of indirect questioning is for the sole purpose of protecting a respondent's privacy and thus enhancing the chances that the respondent would be willing to participate in such a survey and provide honest answers. It is reasonable to assume that on sensitive issues like tax evasion, sexual orientation, gambling, student academic dishonesty, illegal drug use, or criminal activities, people are reluctant to reveal information. Interviewer's assurances that the information furnished would be treated as strictly confidential are just not enough. Even in cases that one agrees to participate in a survey on sensitive issues, there is no guarantee that the information provided is correct. It is very human that people would provide untruthful answers just to be on the safe side. It is for this reason that the need for indirect questioning techniques arises.

Warner (1965) is the first researcher who came up with such a technique termed the Randomized Response Technique (RRT). Assume that by A we denote the sensitive or stigmatizing characteristic. Each person picked up at random is offered a box full of a number of cards identical in shape, size, color, weight, thickness, and in every other possible respect, but a fraction p ($0 < p < 1$, $p \neq 0.5$) of them are marked as A and the rest marked as A^c, the complement of A. The person is requested, outside of view of the interviewer, to randomly draw a card from the box out, after thoroughly shaking it and to truthfully say "Yes" if the mark on the card picked coincides with his/her status about the sensitive characteristic, i.e., to say "Yes" if he/she belongs to the sensitive group and the card picked up is marked A, or if he/she does not have the sensitive attribute and the card picked up is marked as A^c. Otherwise the respondent must respond "No." The respondent is of course not to divulge the card type to the enquirer and he/she is advised to put the card back to the box after truthfully declaring "Yes" or "No" to say if his/her real trait "matches" the card type drawn or "does not match" it. Hopefully the person so addressed is supposed to cooperate because the enquirer cannot be sure if "Yes" is the reply from a person bearing A or bearing the complement A^c as a matter of fact. It is important to emphasize that clear instructions must be given to the participants before they apply any randomized response procedure, or any indirect questioning technique for that matter. In addition, one should make sure that the participants are convinced that the procedure protects their privacy and their status related to the sensitive characteristic. Here we may add that the randomization device does not have to be a box of cards such as the one described above but could be any other device which can be used in such a way so that the respondent responds (with a "Yes" or "No") with probability p to the statement

(I) I have the characteristic A

and with probability $1 - p$ to the statement

(II) I have the characteristic A^c.

Such a device could be a standard deck of cards or even a fair coin or fair die appropriately used. Based on the responses obtained from all the participants, the person in charge of the survey is able to provide estimates for the prevalence of the stigmatizing characteristic as well as other measures associated with it.

Warner's technique has been followed by numerous other procedures. In all such cases, the objective remains the same: To estimate quantities related to sensitive attributes and at the same time to protect the privacy of the participants.

1.2 Real and Hypothetical Examples to Justify the Need for Indirect Methods

In the Netherlands, Scheers (1992), Kerkvliet (1994), van der Heijden and van Gils (1996), van der Heijden, van Gils, Bouts, and Hox (2000), Umesh and Peterson (1991) among others, like Maddala (1983), have been working long in examining efficacies of rival competitive survey techniques of specific nature. Those techniques were aiming at gathering useful data relating to sensitive issues and estimating proportions of people in the communities with propensities to indulge in practicing illegal, immoral, and unlawful practices, or practices considered to be having some cost, for instance not supporting the regime in a dictatorship.

van der Heijden et al. (2000) discuss the following case. From Police files, information was gathered about the people enjoying unemployment benefits while being not eligible. The curiosity was about how many of them would admit, on enquiry, of their complicity in this offensive act. Another couple of stigmatizing habits they considered were students' consumption of marijuana and cheating in examinations. The survey techniques they illustrate as employed are (1) Face-to-Face interviewing by the investigators, (2) Computer-Assisted Self-Interviewing, and (3) RRTs introduced by Warner (1965), the Unrelated Question Randomized Response Model by Abul-Ela, Greenberg, and Horvitz (1967), and Greenberg, Abul-Ela, Simmons, and Horvitz (1969), Kuk's (1990) Randomized Response Technique and the Forced Response Randomized Response Technique introduced by Boruch (1972). In order to improve upon the efficiency levels and also to identify factors that induce truthful answers to queries, they also made use of covariates like age, sex, racial trait, literacy levels, following Maddala (1983) among others.

In a recent study, Dietz et al. (2013) used an RRT approach to estimate the prevalence of cognitive enhancing drug use among university students in Germany. Based on their findings they argue that direct survey techniques used in the past have underestimated the use of those drugs. In a related study, Franke et al. (2013)

by means of the same RRT used in Dietz et al. (2013), estimated the prevalence of pharmacological cognitive enhancement or mood enhancement drugs among surgeons. It is known that surgeons often make use of such drugs in order to combat fatigue, distress and concentration deficits. But it is also known that this particular drug use may lead to addiction and overestimation of the surgeon's own capabilities, thus putting patients at risk.

Kuha and Jackson (2013) analyzed data on the illegal behavior of buying stolen goods. Data were obtained by applying the Item Count Technique with the use of an "item count question" included in the Euro-Justis Survey. The Item Count Technique, to be presented in Chap. 6, seems to be gaining a lot of momentum and it appears to be popular among social survey practitioners.

Karlan and Zinman (2012) have also implemented the Item Count Technique in order to estimate how clients of microfinance institutions spent their loan proceeds, thus providing an application of indirect questioning in the area of economics.

Jan, Jerke, and Krumpal (2012) used the Crosswise Model, one of the so called non randomized response models to measure plagiarism at Swiss and German universities. On the issue of student plagiarism is the paper of Coutts, Jann, Krumpal, and Naeher (2011) where three indirect questioning techniques, the RRT, the Item Count Technique and the Crosswise Model are evaluated for measuring the prevalence of plagiarism in student papers. The academic disintegrity of students and in particular medical students is measured by means of the RRT in Hejri, Zendehdel, Asghari, Fotouhi, and Rashidian (2013).

Ecology and the environment are areas where indirect questioning techniques have found application. In John, Edwards-Jones, Gibbons, and Jones (2010) two indirect questioning techniques, the RRT and the Nominative Technique are presented as methods to estimate the prevalence of rule breaking in conservation. In Blank and Gavin (2009) the RRT is used to estimate the extend of illegal fishing in Northern California.

The prevalence of illegal drug use by professional athletes is not easy to measure by conventional survey research methods. Thus, indirect questioning techniques have been used instead. Striegel, Simon, Hansel, Niess, and Ulrich (2006), Striegel, Ulrich and Simon (2010) and Pitsch, Emrich, and Klein (2007) use the RRT to measure the prevalence of doping among elite athletes. In Chap. 6, we provide model questionnaires for the Item Count Technique which could be used for the same purpose.

In some cases, an opinion expressed even in modern democratic societies might be considered of sensitive or stigmatizing nature. For example a person may have difficulties expressing his/her opinion about an ethnic group or another group (different from his/her own) in the same society. Social scientists find it convenient to employ indirect questioning techniques to gather information on how members of a certain group view another group. Research on racism, sexism or xenophobia may find indirect questioning techniques as an invaluable tool. In a recent study in Germany, described in Krumpal (2012), it is documented that Randomized Response is an effective technique eliciting socially undesirable opinions and provides more accurate prevalence estimates of xenophobia and anti-Semitism than direct questioning.

Quantitative characteristics like number of induced abortion experienced so far by women interviewees, amounts gained or lost in gambling, amounts underreported in income tax returns, amounts surreptitiously earned in excess of legitimate earnings through kickbacks and bribes, numbers of days of drunken driving, amounts spent on items shameful enough to be hidden from the spouses, are some of the quantitative features socially needed to be examined, if actually rampant in a civil society. Many more of course may also be easily named. Indirect questioning tactics seem to be necessary and should be adequately explored by the social scientists indeed.

Not much is known about actual coverage of successfully applied procedures in statistical estimation of parameters relating to quantitative sensitive procedures. However, extensive theoretical research is known to have been carried out over the years to cover such issues. One can mention the work of Greenberg, Kuebler, Abernathy, and Horvitz (1971), Sen (1974), Chaudhuri (1987), Arnab (1995), Singh, Mahmood and Tracy (2001), Bar-Lev, Bobovitch and Boukai (2004), Huang, Lan and Kuo (2006), Saha (2008), Pal (2008), Bouza (2009) and Diana and Perri (2011) among others. Chaudhuri's (2011) monograph can be used as a reference for the case of quantitative sensitive attributes.

Whatever is presented so far in this introductory chapter may appear nebulous. However, we believe that things will become clear and the importance of the methods presented in this monograph will be greatly appreciated by social survey practitioners and mathematical statisticians.

References

Abul-Ela, Abdel-Latif, A., Greenberg, B.G., Horvitz, D.G. (1967). A multi-proportion randomized response model. *Journal of the American Statistical Association*, *62*, 990–1008.

Arnab, R. (1995). Optimal estimation of a finite population total under randomized response surveys. *Statistics*, *27*, 175–180.

Bar-Lev Shaul, K., Bobovitch, E., Boukai, B. (2004). A note on randomized response models for quantitative data. *Metrika*, *60*, 255–260.

Blank, S., & Gavin, M. (2009). The randomized response technique as a tool for estimating non-compliance rates in fisheries: a case study of illegal red abalone (*Haliotis rufescens*) fishing in Northern California. *Environmental Conservation*, *36*, 112–119.

Boruch, R.F. (1972). Relations among statistical methods for assuring confidentiality of social research data. *Social Science Research*, *1*, 403–414.

Bouza, C.N. (2009). Ranked set sampling and randomized response procedures for estimating the mean of a sensitive quantitative character. *Metrika*, *70*, 267–277.

Chaudhuri, A. (1987). Randomized response surveys of finite populations: a unified approach with quantitative data. *Journal of Statistical Planning and Inference*, *15*, 157–165.

Chaudhuri, A. (2011). *Randomized response and indirect questioning techniques in surveys*. Boca Raton: Chapman & Hall, CRC Press, Taylor & Francis Group.

Coutts, E., Jann, B., Ivar, K., Anatol-Fiete, N. (2011). Plagiarism in student papers: prevalence estimates using special techniques for sensitive questions. *Journal of Economics and Statistics, 231*, 749–760.

Diana, G., & Perri, P.F. (2011). A class of estimators for quantitative sensitive data. *Statistical Papers, 52*, 633–650.

Dietz, P., Striegel, H., Franke, G.A., Lieb, K., Simon, P., Ulrich, R. (2013). Randomized response estimates for the 12-month prevalence of cognitive-enhancing drug use in university students. *Pharmacotherapy, 33*, 44–50.

Franke, G.A., Bagusat, C., Dietz, P., Hoffmann, I., Simon, P., Ulrich, R., Lieb, K. (2013). Use of illicit and prescription drugs for cognitive or mood enhancement among surgeons. *MBC Medicine*, doi:10.1186/1741-7015-11-102.

Greenberg, B.G., Abul-Ela, A.-L.A., Simmons, W.R., Horvitz, D.G. (1969). The unrelated question RR model: theoretical framework. *Journal of the American Statistical Association, 64*, 520–539.

Greenberg, B.G., Kuebler, R.R., Abernathy, J.R., Horvitz, D.G. (1971). Application of randomized response technique in obtaining quantitative data. *Journal of the American Statistical Association, 66*, 243–250.

Hejri, M.S., Zendehdel, K., Asghari, F., Fotouhi, A., Rashidian, A. (2013). Academic disintegrity among medical students: a randomized response technique study. *Medical Education, 47*, 144–153.

Huang, K.-C., Lan, C.-H., Kuo, M.-P. (2006). Estimation of sensitive quantitative characteristics in randomized response sampling. *Journal of Statistics and Management Systems, 9*, 27–35.

Jann, B., Jerke, J., Krumpal, I. (2012). Asking sensitive questions using the crosswise model. An experimental survey measuring plagiarism. *Public Opinion Quarterly, 76*, 32–49.

John, F.A.V. St., Edwards-Jones, G., Gibbons, J.M., Jones, J.P.G. (2010). Testing novel methods for assessing rule breaking in conservation. *Biological Conservation, 143*, 1025–1030.

Karlan, D.S., & Zinman, J. (2012). List randomization for sensitive behavior: an application for measuring use of loan proceeds. *Journal of Developmental Economics, 98*, 71–75.

Kerkvliet, J. (1994). Estimating a logit model with randomized data: the case of cocaine use. *Australian Journal of Statistics, 36*, 9–20.

Kuha, J., & Jackson, J. (2013). The item count method for sensitive survey questions: modelling criminal behavior. *Journal of the Royal Statistical Society: Series C (Applied Statistics)*, forthcoming.

Kuk Anthony, Y.C. (1990). Asking sensitive questions indirectly. *Biometrika, 77*, 436–438.

Krumpal, I. (2012). Estimating the prevalence of xenophobia and anti-Semitism in Germany: a comparison of randomized response and direct questioning. *Social Science Research, 41*, 1387–1403.

Maddala, G.S. (1983). *Limited dependent and qualitative variables in econometrics.* New York: Cambridge University Press.

Pal, S. (2008). Unbiasedly estimating the total of a stigmatizing variable from a complex survey on permitting options for direct or randomized responses. *Statistical Papers, 49*, 157–164.

Pitsch, W., Emrich, E., Klein, M. (2007). Doping in elite sports in Germany: results on www survey. *European Journal of Sport and Society, 4*, 89–102.

Saha, A. (2008). A randomized response technique for quantitative data under unequal probability sampling. *Journal of Statistical Theory and Practice, 2*, 589–596.

Scheers, N.J. (1992). A review of randomized response techniques. *Measurement and Evaluation in Counseling and Development, 25*, 27–41.

Sen, P.K. (1974). On unbiased estimation for randomized response models. *Journal of the American Statistical Association, 69*, 997–1001.

Singh, S., Mahmood, M., Tracy, D.S. (2001). Estimation of mean and variance of stigmatized quantitative variable using distinct units in randomized response sampling. *Statistical Papers, 42*, 403–411.

Striegel, H., Simon, P., Hansel, J., Niess, A.M., Ulrich, R. (2006). Doping and drug use in elite sports: an analysis using the randomized technique. *Medicine and Science in Sports and Exercise, 38*, 247.

References

Striegel, H., Ulrich, R., Simon, P. (2010). Randomized response estimates for doping and illicit drug use in elite athletes. *Drug and Alcohol Dependence, 106,* 230–232.

Umesh, U.N., & Peterson, R.A. (1991). A critical evaluation of the randomized response method. *Social Methods Research, 20,* 104–138.

van der Heijden, P.G.M., & van Gils, G. (1996). Some logistic regression models for randomized response data. In *Proceedings of the 11th International Workshop on Statistical Modelling,* Orvieto, Italy.

van der Heijden, P.G.M., van Gils, G., Bouts, J., Hox, J. (2000). A comparison of randomized response, Computer assisted Self Interview, and Face to Face Direct Questioning; eliciting sensitive information in the context of welfare and unemployment benefits. *Sociological Methods and Research, 28,* 505–537.

Warner Stanley, L. (1965). Randomized Response: a survey technique for eliminating evasive answer bias. *Journal of the American Statistical Association, 60,* 63–69.

Chapter 2
Specification of Qualitative and Quantitative Parameters Demanding Estimation

Abstract In this chapter the basic and rudimentary aspects of sample surveys for finite populations are presented in a compact way. The concepts of population, sample, sampling design, survey data, estimating finite population parameters of interest and consequent errors and their control will be explained and detailed illustrations will be provided. The theory to address general issues will be explained first. Then the need for modification to cover the case of sensitive issues and how to do that will be explained. It will be clearly shown how in a general situation one may handle indirectly procured observations to estimate parameters of interest and also derive estimated measures of accuracy. Sophisticated theoretical details will be presented only in brief. Finally in this chapter we put emphasis on the fact that any probability sampling design may be employed for the purpose of estimating parameters related to stigmatizing characteristics.

2.1 Introduction

A labeled finite population of identifiable individuals, each bearing real numbered values including zero and one is supposed to be surveyed through sampling and ascertaining sample-wise values to estimate certain parameters. Specifically, we take up the case of individual human beings, some of whom bear sensitive, rather stigmatizing features. A way out is needed to successfully gather individual values for respective people sampled so as to estimate proportions of a community bearing such sensitive features or the total value for a stigmatizing characteristic borne collectively by the members of a community.

As the title of this monograph announces it is avowedly one on survey sampling. So, we are under an obligation to tell our readers certain basic and rudimentary aspects of sample surveys.

By $U = (1, \ldots, i, \ldots, N)$ we shall mean a survey population. It refers to a known finite number N of individuals labeled for identification uniquely by i which stands for the label 1 through N, each denoting just one of these N units. Each unit i bears a value y_i for a real variable y, $i = 1, \ldots, N$. Thus the vector $\underline{Y} = (y_1, \ldots, y_i, \ldots, y_N)$ is defined on U. Then

$$Y = \sum_{i=1}^{N} y_i, \quad \bar{Y} = \frac{Y}{N}, \quad S^2 = \frac{1}{N-1} \sum_{i=1}^{N} (y_i - \bar{Y})^2$$

are some of the parameters of common interest related to $\underline{Y}$. The quantities Y and $\bar{Y}$ are usually required to be estimated, called, respectively, the total and mean of y related to U. The quantity S^2 is the population variance. For estimation, a sample s of elements of U is required to be chosen with a pre-assigned probability $p(s)$ according to a suitable probability design or design in brief for simplicity, say, such that $0 \le p(s) \le 1$ for every sample s that may be selected from U. The number of units in s, say, n is called the size of s, just as N is the size of the population U. On choosing a sample, the values of y for the units in s, that is, y_i for $i \in s$ are to be ascertained by dint of an actual sample survey. On gathering the survey data

$$d = (s, y_i | i \in s),$$

an estimator for Y may be employed as $t = t(d)$, usually with the properties

$$E_p(t) = \sum_s p(s) t(d) = Y$$

and

$$M_p(t) = E_p(t - Y)^2 = \sum_s p(s)(t(d) - Y)^2,$$

being suitably small. The quantity $M_p(t)$ is called the mean square error, and E_p denotes the expectation operator with respect to the sampling design p. Such a t is called an estimator for Y with its error $(t - Y)$ such that $M_p(t)$ is suitably under control. If K is a pre-assigned positive number, noting that we may write

$$M_p(t) = \sum_1 p(s)(t(d) - Y)^2 + \sum_2 p(s)(t(d) - Y)^2 \ge K^2 P\left[s : |t(d) - Y| \ge K\right],$$

where $\sum_1$ is the sum over those samples for which $|t(d) - Y| \ge K$ and $\sum_2$ that over the complementary set of possible samples, it follows that

$$P\left[t(d) - K < Y < t(d) + K\right] \ge 1 - \frac{M_p(t)}{K^2}.$$

The quantity

$$B_p(t) = E_p(t - Y)$$

2.1 Introduction

is called the bias of t in estimating Y and

$$\sigma_p(t) = +\sqrt{\sigma_p^2(t)} = +\sqrt{V_p(t)}$$

is the standard error of t, where

$$V_p(t) = E_p(t - E_p(t))^2,$$

is the variance of t. Now

$$M_p(t) = V_p(t) + B_p^2(t).$$

Consequently, by taking $K = \lambda \sigma_p(t)$, with $\lambda > 0$, it follows that

$$P\left[t(d) - \lambda\sigma_p(t) < Y < t(d) + \lambda\sigma_p(t)\right] \geq \left(1 - \frac{1}{\lambda^2}\right) - \frac{1}{\lambda^2}\left(\frac{|B_p(t)|}{\sigma_p(t)}\right)^2.$$

If t is chosen to be unbiased for Y, then

$$P\left[Y \in \left(t(d) - \lambda\sigma_p(t),\ t(d) + \lambda\sigma_p(t)\right)\right] \geq \left(1 - \frac{1}{\lambda^2}\right).$$

The interval

$$t(d) \pm \lambda\sigma_p(t)$$

is called a confidence interval (CI) for Y with a confidence coefficient (CC) of at least

$$\left(1 - \frac{1}{\lambda^2}\right).$$

So, it is desirable to employ an unbiased estimator t for Y with $B_p(t) = 0$ and a small variance because in that case one may derive a confidence interval based on $t(d)$ with a small width equal to $2\lambda\sigma_p(t)$. For example, a choice of $\lambda = 3$ will yield

$$t(d) \pm 3\sigma_p(t)$$

as a confidence interval with a confidence coefficient of at least as high as $8/9$. Neyman (1934) gave us this gift for survey sampling extending Chebyshev's inequality in probability theory.

Unfortunately however, as Basu (1971) has shown, unless a census, i.e., a complete enumeration of a survey population is undertaken, no sampling design admits an unbiased estimator for a finite population total ensuring a minimum value for its variance, uniformly for every $\underline{Y} = (y_1, \ldots, y_i, \ldots, y_N)$ assigning any real number to each coordinate of $\underline{Y}$. Following Godambe (1955), let us restrict to the use of an estimator $t = t(d)$ of the form

$$t = t_b = \sum_{i \in s} y_i b_{si}$$

such that b_{si} are numbers free of $\underline{Y}$ subject to the restriction

$$\sum_{s \ni i} p(s) b_{si} = 1, \ \forall \ i \in U, \qquad (2.1)$$

where $\sum_{s \ni i}$ means summation over all samples s which contain the unit labeled i. The condition given by (2.1) is necessary as well as sufficient to render t_b unbiased for Y. Unfortunately again, Godambe (1955) has shown that in the class of all such estimators for Y of the form t_b as above, called the class of Homogeneous Linear Unbiased Estimators (HLUE), no one exists with a Uniformly Minimum Variance (UMV), so long as it is based on a "general" class of designs p. Godambe (1955) did not specify what he meant by his "general" class. But Hege (1965) and Hanurav (1966) independently showed that a general class of designs called Uniclustered Class of Designs (UCD) exists for which the above negative result does not hold. A design p belonging to a UCD is a design such that for any two samples s_1 and s_2 with $p(s_1) > 0$ and $p(s_2) > 0$ either

1. $s_1 \cap s_2$ is empty, i.e., s_2 does not intersect with s_1

or

2. $s_1 \sim s_2$, i.e., every unit of s_1 is in s_2 and vice versa.

Thus, Godambe's (1955) above celebrated nonexistence result is valid only for non uni-cluster-designs (NUCD).

Hege (1965), Hanurav (1966), and quite elegantly Lanke (1975) have shown that a UCD admits a UMV estimator for Y in the HLUE class. Importantly, this UMV estimator in the class HLUE for Y is of the form

$$t_{HT} = \sum_{i \in s} \frac{y_i}{\pi_i},$$

where $\pi_i = \sum_{s \ni i} p(s)$. The estimator t_{HT} is given by Horvitz and Thompson (1952). The quantity π_i is called the "inclusion-probability" of a unit i in U being included in a sample chosen according to a design p. It may be noted that there is no problem in taking π_i into the denominator in t_{HT} because a well-known fact in "Survey Sampling Theory" is that a "Necessary and Sufficient Condition" that an unbiased estimator for Y may exist is that

$$\pi_i > 0, \ \forall \ i \in U.$$

See Chaudhuri (2010) for details.

2.1 Introduction

Most of the estimators for Y used in practice are in the HLUE class. If we add the terms b_s to t_b such that b_s is free of $\underline{Y}$ and $E_p(b_s) = 0$, then we get

$$t_L = b_s + \sum_{i \in s} y_i b_{si},$$

a nonhomogeneous Linear Unbiased Estimator for Y, the LUE class. No estimator for Y outside this LUE class is ever put into practice except that the unbiasedness conditions

$$E_p(b_s) = 0 \text{ and } \sum_{s \ni i} p(s) b_{si} = 1 \ \forall \ i \in U$$

are often relaxed. The estimators t_L, t_b for Y are admitted provided the quantities $B_p(t_L)$ and $B_p(t_b)$ are numerically small enough, at least for large n. The HLUEs for Y and in particular the Horvitz and Thompson's (1952) estimator, say, are the most popular. Added to them, Hajek's (1971) ratio estimator

$$t_H = \frac{X \sum_{i \in s}(y_i/\pi_i)}{\sum_{i \in s}(x_i/\pi_i)},$$

where x_i are known (positive) values of a variable x, highly and positively correlated with y and where $X = \sum_{i=1}^{N} x_i$, mostly exhaust the popular estimators for Y. This ratio estimator with its denominator even as a random variable as s is so, is yet in Godambe's class of linear homogeneous estimators for Y because this t_H is linear in the y_i's and there is no term in it free of $\underline{Y}$ and cannot be nonhomogeneous.

We consider it important to observe:

$$V_p(t_b) = E_p(t_b - Y)^2 = \sum_i y_i^2 C_i + \sum_i \sum_{j, j \neq i} y_i y_j C_{ij},$$

where

$$C_i = \sum_{s \ni i} p(s) b_{si}^2 - 1$$

and

$$C_{ij} = \sum_{s \ni i, j} p(s) b_{si} b_{sj} - 1.$$

The quantity

$$v_p(t_b) = \sum_{i \in s} y_i^2 C_{si} + \sum_{i \in s} \sum_{j \in s, j \neq i} y_i y_j C_{sij}$$

is an unbiased estimator for $V_p(t_b)$ on choosing C_{si} and C_{sij}'s as free of $\underline{Y}$ subject to the conditions

$$\sum_s p(s)C_{si} = C_i, \ \forall \ i \in U$$

and

$$\sum_s p(s)C_{sij} = C_{ij}, \ \forall \ i, j \in U, \ i \neq j.$$

More generally, on choosing

$$\underline{W} = (w_1, \ldots, w_i, \ldots, w_N), \ w_i \neq 0 \ \forall \ i \in U$$

as a vector of pre-assigned constants, it follows that

$$V_p(t_b) = -\sum_i \sum_{j,j>i} d_{ij} w_i w_j \left(\frac{y_i}{w_i} - \frac{y_j}{w_j}\right)^2 + \sum_i \frac{y_i^2}{w_i} \alpha_i,$$

where

$$d_{ij} = E_p(b_{si}I_{si} - 1)(b_{sj}I_{sj} - 1),$$

$$I_{si} = \begin{cases} 1 & \text{if } s \ni i \\ 0 & \text{otherwise} \end{cases}$$

and

$$\alpha_i = \sum_j d_{ij} w_j.$$

Writing

$$\pi_{ij} = \sum_{s \ni i,j} p(s)$$

as the probability of i and j ($i \neq j$) both included in a sample chosen according to a design p and in addition supposing $\pi_{ij} > 0 \ \forall \ i \neq j$ and of course $\pi_i > 0 \ \forall \ i \in U$ to get t_b unbiased for Y, one may get an unbiased estimator for $V_p(t_b)$ as

$$v_p(t_b) = -\sum_{i \in s} \sum_{j \in s, j>i} d_{sij} w_i w_j \left(\frac{y_i}{w_i} - \frac{y_j}{w_j}\right)^2 + \sum_{i \in s} \frac{y_i^2 \alpha_i}{w_i \pi_i},$$

2.1 Introduction

on taking the d_{sij}'s as free of $\underline{Y}$ subject to

$$\sum_s p(s) d_{sij} = d_{ij}, \forall\, i \neq j,$$

e.g., as $d_{sij} = (d_{ij}/\pi_{ij})\ \forall\, i \neq j$ in s and in U. In particular,

$$V_p(t_{HT}) = \sum_{i=1}^N y_i^2 \frac{1-\pi_i}{\pi_i} + \sum_i \sum_{j,j\neq i} y_i y_j \frac{\pi_{ij} - \pi_i \pi_j}{\pi_i \pi_j}$$

and

$$v_p(t_{HT}) = \sum_{i\in s} y_i^2 \frac{1-\pi_i}{\pi_i}\frac{I_{si}}{\pi_i} + \sum_{i\in s}\sum_{j\in s, j\neq i} y_i y_j \left(\frac{\pi_{ij} - \pi_i \pi_j}{\pi_i \pi_j}\right)\frac{I_{sij}}{\pi_{ij}}.$$

Also, alternatively,

$$V_p(t_{HT}) = \sum_i \sum_{j,j>i} (\pi_i \pi_j - \pi_{ij})\left(\frac{y_i}{\pi_i} - \frac{y_j}{\pi_j}\right)^2 + \sum \frac{y_i^2}{w_i}\beta_i,$$

taking $w_i = \pi_i$ and writing

$$\beta_i = 1 + \frac{1}{\pi_i}\sum_{j,j\neq i}\pi_{ij} - \sum_{i=1}^N \pi_i$$

and an unbiased estimator for $V_p(t_{HT})$ is

$$v_p(t_{HT}) = \sum_{i\in s}\sum_{j\in s, j>i}\left(\frac{\pi_i \pi_j - \pi_{ij}}{\pi_{ij}}\right)\left(\frac{y_i}{\pi_i} - \frac{y_j}{\pi_j}\right)^2 + \sum \frac{y_i^2}{\pi_i}\beta_i \frac{I_{si}}{\pi_i}.$$

It should be noted that if every sample s with $p(s) > 0$ has a constant number of distinct units in it, then $\beta_i = 0$. Consequently $V_p(t_{HT})$ and $v_p(t_{HT})$ take the familiar forms due to Yates and Grundy (1953) namely,

$$V_{YG} = \sum_i \sum_{j,j>i} (\pi_i \pi_j - \pi_{ij})\left(\frac{y_i}{\pi_i} - \frac{y_j}{\pi_j}\right)^2$$

and

$$v_{YG} = \sum_{i\in s}\sum_{j\in s, j>i} (\pi_i \pi_j - \pi_{ij})\left(\frac{y_i}{\pi_i} - \frac{y_j}{\pi_j}\right)^2 \frac{1}{\pi_{ij}},$$

respectively.

Remark 2.1. As in Chaudhuri's (2011) textbook, the spirit in which this monograph has been written demands a reader/researcher to feel comfortable with randomized response data (and data produced by other indirect questioning techniques to be illustrated in this monograph), being procured from sampled persons in specifically prescribed ways no matter how selected, so that inferences may be drawn and suitably assessed on choosing the samples in desirable ways, with equal or unequal selection probabilities, with or without replacement. In a vast majority of the space covered in publications on data gathered by indirect questioning techniques, samples are chosen by Simple Random Sampling with Replacement (SRSWR). In such a case, the simple arithmetic mean of suitably transformed individual observations is employed to unbiasedly estimate $\bar{Y}$ and variances and variance estimators are derived along the standard SRSWR procedure. In very few cases, when y is just a binary variable taking on the values 0 and 1 representing an innocuous and stigmatizing feature respectively borne by a person, samples are not chosen by simple random sampling with replacement.

Chaudhuri's (2011) textbook is claimed to offer a quick appreciation of our approach set forth here.

2.2 Estimating Parameters

We shall consider only two possibilities:

(I) Every y_i is either 1, implying a person labeled i bears a stigmatizing characteristic or attribute, say, A, or 0 implying the i-th person's attribute being A^c, i.e., the complement of A, meaning that the person does not have the stigmatizing characteristic; our problem is to estimate $\bar{Y}$ to be denoted by θ, the proportion in a community U bearing A.
(II) Every y_i is a real number and our aim is to estimate the population total Y.

From our treatment in Sect. 2.1 an outline of a possible procedure readily follows. As a measure of accuracy in estimation we recommend evaluating the coefficient of variation (CV) as

$$CV = 100 \frac{+\sqrt{v_p(t)}}{t}$$

for a choice of t as illustrated.

Since t_H is not unbiased for Y we need to consider only its Mean Square Error (MSE)

$$M(t_H) = E_p \left[X \frac{t_{HT}(y)}{t_{HT}(x)} - Y \right]^2$$

2.2 Estimating Parameters

approximately taken as, on assuming n quite large,

$$M(t_H) = X^2 V_p(t_{HT})\,|_{\underline{Y}=\underline{Y}-R\underline{X}},$$

where $R = (Y/X)$ and recognizing $V_p(t_{HT})$ as a formula for $V_p\left(\sum_{i\in s}(y_i/\pi_i)\right)$ evaluated with y_i replaced by $d_i = y_i - Rx_i$, $i \in U$. By $t(y), t(x)$ we mean an estimator for Y using y_i, $i \in s$ and the same one with x_i, $i \in s$. Then a plausible estimator for $M(t_H)$ is taken as

$$m(t_H) = [t_{HT}(x)]^2 v_p(t_{HT})\,|_{\underline{Y}=\underline{Y}-\hat{R}\underline{X}},$$

writing $\hat{R} = t_{HT}(y)/t_{HT}(x)$ and in the formula for $v_p(t_{HT})$ taking $y_i - \hat{R}x_i$ throughout for $i \in s$ in lieu of y_i, $i \in s$. Chaudhuri (2010) may be consulted for clarification. Needless to mention the coefficient of variation for t_H will be taken as

$$CV(t_H) = 100\frac{+\sqrt{m(t_H)}}{t_H}$$

as an approximation, assuming n large enough.

All these are applicable only provided y_i is available for i in s. But in the situations of our interest, they are not. An investigator, out of sheer delicacy hesitates to ask a respondent to disclose his/her value on a sensitive variable. Even if he/she dares, a respondent is likely to refuse or hide the truth giving an untruthful or misleading response.

In the subsequent chapters we shall narrate diverse procedures to tackle this situation. The gist is that we may point out at this stage that by a suitable "random" mechanism we claim we may gather observations r_i, "independently" across i in s, such that

$$E_R(r_i) = y_i,\ \forall\, i \in U,$$

where E_R denotes a generic expectation operator with respect to such a random mechanism employed.

In situation (I) when y_i takes on either the value zero or one only,

$$\begin{aligned}V_R(r_i) &= E_R(r_i - E_R(r_i))^2 \\ &= E_R(r_i^2) - y_i^2 \\ &= E_R(r_i^2) - y_i \\ &= E_R[r_i(r_i - 1)] \\ &= V_i,\end{aligned}$$

say, writing V_R as the generic variance operator for the variance calculation with respect to the random mechanism mentioned above. Then $v_i = r_i(r_i - 1)$ provides an unbiased estimator for V_i.

In situation (II) we shall be able to show for our illustrated applications of the "random" mechanisms that for real y_i, an unbiased estimator r_i will be derivable independently across i in s so that $E_R(r_i) = y_i, \forall i \in U$; moreover, generically, $V_R(r_i)$ will be shown to be of the form

$$V_i = V_R(r_i) = \alpha_i y_i^2 + \beta_i y_i + \Psi_i$$

with $\alpha_i, \beta_i, \Psi_i$ as known constants and consequently,

$$v_i = \frac{1}{1+\alpha_i}(\alpha_i r_i^2 + \beta_i r_i + \Psi_i)$$

is an unbiased estimator for $V_R(r_i)$. Then, it will follow that given $t_b = t_b(d)$ with $E_p(t) = Y$, so that $\sum_{s \ni i} p(s) b_{si} = 1$,

$$V_p(t_b) = \sum y_i^2 C_i + \sum_i \sum_{j, j \neq i} y_i y_j C_{ij}$$

and

$$v_p(t_b) = \sum_{i \in s} y_i^2 C_{si} + \sum_{i \in s} \sum_{j \in s, j \neq i} y_i y_j C_{sij},$$

one might employ, writing $\underline{R} = (r_1, \ldots, r_i, \ldots, r_N)$

$$e_b = t_b \mid_{\underline{Y}=\underline{R}} = \sum r_i b_{si},$$

$$E(e_b) = E_p E_R(e_b) = E_R E_p(e_b) = Y,$$

$$V(e_b) = E_p V_R(e_b) + V_p E_R(e_b) = E_R V_p(e_b) + V_R E_p(e_b).$$

Then

$$v_1(e_b) = v_p(e_b) \mid_{\underline{Y}=\underline{R}} + \sum_{i \in s} v_i b_{si}$$

and

$$v_2(e_b) = v_p(e_b) \mid_{\underline{Y}=\underline{R}} + \sum_{i \in s} v_i (b_{si}^2 - C_{si})$$

will both satisfy

$$E(v_1(e_b)) = V(e_b) = E(v_2(e_b)),$$

where

$$E = E_p E_R = E_R E_p$$

and

$$V = E_p V_R + V_p E_R = E_R V_p + V_R E_p.$$

Thus, it is clear how in a general situation one may handle indirectly procured observations to estimate θ and Y and also derive estimated measures of accuracy in estimation, in terms of coefficients of variation (CV). As a rule of thumb, we could consider an estimate as excellent if for an estimated CV, it is true that $CV \leq 10\%$, as satisfactory if $10\% < CV \leq 20\%$, as acceptable if $20\% < CV \leq 30\%$ and as unacceptable if $CV > 30\%$.

2.3 How to Sample?

Any probability sampling scheme depending upon available resources may be employed. Chaudhuri's (2010) may be utilized as a companion to take care of this for simplicity. Chaudhuri's (2011) monograph may be utilized in gathering guidelines in their utilization in estimation.

2.4 How to Gather Sensitive Data?

We may recognize that facing a given situation, an investigator may consider an issue to be sensitive enough so that an indirect questioning technique may seem to be necessary. For this, requisite procedures are narrated in subsequent chapters. If the investigator deems it doubtful if he/she should go for a direct or indirect questioning, then also appropriate procedures may be followed as given in later chapters. Corresponding estimation procedures are also set forth in the right places in detail.

References

Basu, D. (1971). An essay on the logical foundations of survey sampling, Part 1. In V.P. Godambe, D.A. Sprott (Eds.), *Foundations of statistical inference* (pp. 203–242). Toronto: Holt, Rinehart & Winston.
Chaudhuri, A. (2010). *Essentials of survey sampling*. New Delhi: Prentice Hall of India.
Chaudhuri, A. (2011). *Randomized response and indirect questioning techniques in surveys*. Boca Raton: Chapman & Hall, CRC Press, Taylor & Francis Group.

Godambe, V.P. (1955). A unified theory of sampling from finite populations. *Journal of the Royal Statistical Society: Series B, 17,* 269–278.
Hajek, J. (1971). Comment on a paper by Basu. In V.P. Godambe, D.A. Sprott (Eds.), *Foundations of statistical inference* (pp. 203–242). Toronto: Holt, Rinehart and Winston.
Hanurav, T.V. (1966). Some aspects of unified sampling theory. *Sankhya, Series A, 28,* 175–204.
Hege, V.S. (1965). Sampling designs which admit uniformly minimum unbiased estimators. *Calcutta Statistical Association Bulletin, 14,* 160–162.
Horvitz, D.G., & Thompson, D.J. (1952). A generalization of sampling without replacement from finite universe. *Journal of Americal Statistical Association, 47,* 663–685.
Lanke, J. (1975). *Some contributions to the theory of survey sampling.* Ph. D. Thesis, University of Lund, Lund, Sweden.
Neyman, J. (1934). On the two different aspects of the representative method: the method of stratified sampling and the method of purposive selection. *Journal of the Royal Statistical Society: Series B, 97,* 199–214.
Yates, F., & Grundy, P.M. (1953). Selection without replacement from within strata with probability proportional to size. *Journal of the Royal Statistical Society: Series B, 15,* 253–261.

Chapter 3
Various Indirect Questioning Techniques

Abstract It will be first emphasized that no matter how a person is selected to be in the sample, an indirect procedure may be adopted to endeavor to gather sensitive data from him/her in deriving sensible estimators for population parameters along with estimated measures of their accuracies. This chapter offers a preview of the indirect questioning techniques that will be presented in subsequent chapters in more detail. The broad and rich class of Randomized Response Techniques and their rationale are presented first. Then three more techniques are discussed briefly, the Item Count Technique, the Nominative Technique, and The Three Card Method along with their rationales. The chapter ends with previews of two of the most recent indirect questioning techniques, the general class of Non Randomized Models which includes techniques where no randomization device is needed and the method of Surveying with Negative Questions where questions are asked in a negative way so that a respondent can provide one of many possible answers.

3.1 Introduction

A major breakthrough in this monograph following Chaudhuri (2001a,b, 2011) more comprehensively) is that we intend to emphasize that in order to gather relevant data on sensitive items of information it is important to adopt indirect questioning techniques from persons sampled, no matter how they happen to be selected. Given the data realized and at hand, it is of our concern to estimate mainly two types of parameters. They are, for a given community whence a sample is drawn, the proportion of people bearing a sensitive characteristic, generically denoted as A when it is an attribute and alternatively the total of the values of a quantitative variable which is stigmatizing like, for example, the amounts of money earned by gambling. First we illustrate how personal data on sensitive issues may be gathered from sampled respondents without a direct query but by a specific indirect way. Then we discuss how such data are to be manipulated to yield plausible estimators for the parameters noted above along with their measures of accuracy.

Warner (1965) was the first to publish an innovative technique to procure responses from selected people relating to immoral, illegal, or unpopular personal issues of stigmatizing nature by a certain indirect type. The resulting response is known as a Randomized Response (RR) rather than a Direct Response (DR). The reason is that a respondent is requested to implement an elementary random trial and report "Yes" or "No" depending on either of two possible outcomes observed to occur for this trial relating to bearing either a sensitive characteristic A or its complement A^c. This seminal work spawned a huge literature on Randomized Response Techniques (RRTs). Though an enthusiasm became well spread, criticisms against its efficacy became rampant too. In consequence, other alternative indirect questioning techniques emerged. One is the "Item Count Technique" (ICT). Here a sampled person is requested to read a list of statements, count how many of them are applicable to him/her, and report only the number of items applicable. In an independently drawn second sample, each participant is requested to read a list of statements which contains the exact same statements as the list presented to the first sample plus a statement related to the stigmatizing characteristic. As before, the person reports only the number of statements which are applicable to him/her.

Another indirect questioning technique is known as the "Nominative Technique" (NT) in which a sampled person is requested to report about one or more acquaintances as to whether they bear a sensitive attribute but he/she is not required to reveal whether he/she personally belongs to the stigmatizing group.

"The Three Card Method" (TCM) is also an alternative indirect questioning technique to be explained in Sect. 3.5.

Another indirect questioning technique to enquire about sensitive characteristics we cover in this monograph is given the name "Non Randomized Response (NRR) Approach." Tian, Yu, Tang, and Geng (2007), Yu, Tian, and Tang (2008), Tan, Tian, and Tang (2009), and Christofides (2009) have so far substantially contributed to Non-Randomized Response Techniques (NRRT) to be elaborated in Sect. 3.6 of the present chapter. Each of these four publications confines to sample selection exclusively by Simple Random Sampling With Replacement (SRSWR) alone. We shall discuss how they may be extended to cover unequal probability sample selection as well.

The final indirect questioning technique to be described in this monograph is a relatively new technique introduced by Esponda (2006) and further developed by Esponda and Guerrero (2009). This technique makes use of negative questions in surveys of human populations and that is why originally the technique is described under the term "Negative Surveys."

3.2 Randomized Response Technique: Its Rationale

It is often very difficult for a researcher to ask questions related to stigmatizing secrets. Even if he/she dares to ask such questions, cooperation from sample people is in doubt. In case people agree to participate in such a survey, usually misleading

3.2 Randomized Response Technique: Its Rationale

and untruthful answers are given. But social research often demands serviceable assessments about extents of incidence and prevalence rates of immoral, unlawful, unpopular, or stigmatizing practices perpetrated by people in various communities. One way out of this difficulty is provided by the celebrated technique of randomized response graciously introduced by Warner (1965). Warner's innovative approach has motivated numerous researchers to further develop RRTs offering many improvements and generalizations. It is a fact that Warner's paper has created a separate field of research activity.

To estimate for a community the proportion of people bearing a stigmatizing characteristic (denoted by the symbol A), like addiction to marijuana consumption or cheating in Income Tax Returns, a sampled person is requested to execute a random experiment. Without divulging the outcome of the random experiment, a sampled person is requested to give out a response from which it is not possible to ascertain whether the person bears A or its complement A^c, say. But it is possible statistically to derive a plausible estimate, on analyzing the bunch of randomized responses thus collectively gathered, for the required proportion bearing A. It is hoped that the privacy of the person responding is securely protected. The actual procedure in estimation along with an estimated measure of accuracy of the estimator derived is of course open for verification to the respondents. A knowledgeable respondent is fully provided the freedom to judge how far the randomized response may distort the probability of a person to bear A "before" the randomized response, compared to what it is "after"-wards. Furthermore, anticipating that a feature "A" deemed stigmatizing by the researcher may actually be held as quite "innocuous" by a respondent, methods have been developed so as to offer a respondent an opportunity to opt either to

1. give out a direct response about bearing A, or
2. apply the RRT preferred without being required to divulge the option actually exercised.

The literature presents a lion's share of the methods with SRSWR of the respondents. But Chaudhuri (2001a,b, 2011) has shown how estimating A does not need a simple random sample with replacement in estimation; any sampling scheme with positive inclusion probability for every member in the community is enough; to measure accuracy in estimation it is enough in addition to assign positive inclusion probability to every distinct pair of different members in the population. If the parameter of interest is the total for the values of a sensitive variable like expenses on alcoholism, treatment of AIDS, gain or loss in gambling, money earned from clandestine sources, etc., then also procedures are available for procuring randomized responses relating to quantitative variables of interest so as to produce serviceable estimates for such totals along with estimated measures of accuracy in estimation. General sampling schemes are usable in such an estimation. Chaudhuri (2011) provides a store of a substantial body of source materials.

3.3 Item Count Technique: Its Rationale

RRTs are adversely criticized mainly on the following counts:

1. They demand too much active cooperation and understanding from the respondents and too much time,
2. face-to-face interview is a must for generation of responses,
3. repeated responses once the survey is over are difficult to come by,
4. it is difficult to dispel respondent's suspicions about clever manipulative cooking of the raw material gathered by the researcher,
5. the use of a randomization device is sometimes considered as a gimmick and often is laughed at, and
6. there is a consequent tendency for declining participation by potential respondents.

Hence alternatives to randomized response were sought. The "ICT" first emerged through the efforts of Miller, Cisin, and Harrel (1986). To one sample taken first, a list of G ($G > 1$) innocuous items is presented. To a second independently taken sample, a list is presented which, in addition to the G innocuous items, contains one more item related to the stigmatizing characteristic. The first sample yields an estimate for the mean number out of the G items that apply positively for the people in the community. The second sample yields a second estimate for the mean number out of the $(G + 1)$ items that apply to the same community of people. Now, the second estimate minus the first rationally provides an estimate of the proportion of the people bearing the $(G + 1)$-st, i.e., the only sensitive item of the researcher's choice. The three authors named above only considered SRSWR in this method. Chapter 6 will show how and with what modifications this method extends to unequal probability design. Various versions of the ICT are available so that the privacy of participants is better protected. In addition, the technique can be modified so that estimation of quantitative sensitive characteristics is also possible. The various versions of the ICT are also presented in Chap. 6.

3.4 Nominative Technique: Its Rationale

In "Essentials of Survey Sampling" Chaudhuri (2010) has narrated his version of "Network Sampling." In it the aim is to estimate the mean of a qualitative variable for a population of individuals called "Observation Units" (OU). Neither the total number nor a "Frame" for these observation units is available to facilitate sample selection and/or parameter estimation. But it is possible to establish a "link" with these observation units of a second collection of objects or individuals called "Selection Units" (SU). The total number and frame for these selection units, then a "Network" may be conceived of and constructed, linking the selection units and the observation units. This may then be exploited to estimate parameters for the observation units.

In order to estimate the proportion θ of people in a community bearing a sensitive attribute A, on gathering relevant sensitive data by indirect questioning, not by means of a randomized response device, Miller (1985) introduced a new method called the "Nominative Method." In it, from a relevant community constituting a population, a SRSWR is chosen and every sampled person is requested to identify the number of his/her acquainted persons known to bear the stigmatizing attribute A. By exploiting the Network Sampling technique and its analogous link with Miller's ideas, Chaudhuri and Christofides (2008) showed how Miller's ideas may be exploited to estimate θ on taking a sample by a suitably general scheme. Details are given in Chap. 6.

3.5 The Three Card Method: Its Rationale

Droitcour, Larson, and Scheuren (2001) gave this method using three independent samples, in each of which, a person is given three separate boxes with three cards bearing identification about characteristics, namely the sensitive one as A and the innocuous ones like B, C, and D, say. Each sampled person is to randomly choose one of the three boxes and announce the box number only. From this response Droitcour et al. (2001) show that it is possible to unbiasedly estimate the proportion of people bearing A. But the theory demands restriction to SRSWR only as per the original method. Chaudhuri and Christofides (2008) extended it to general sampling schemes. Details follow in Chap. 6.

3.6 Non Randomized Models

One of the main disadvantages of RRTs is the use of a randomization device. In some cases participants are having difficulties in using correctly the randomization device, no matter how simple that device may be. In many cases, participants are suspicious about the use of the device. They are not really convinced that their anonymity and privacy is really protected, especially, if the device is provided by the interviewer. As a result, untruthful responses are to be expected, thus, in essence eliminating the gains of using an indirect questioning technique instead of a direct answer survey. To overcome this difficulty, some techniques, termed non randomized techniques offer an alternative. Although called non randomized, they could be called device-free techniques because no randomization device is needed. However, that does not mean that no randomization takes place. In some cases, an implicit randomization is performed. For example in Christofides (2009) a randomization is done based on the sensitive characteristic and the participant provides a "Yes" or "No" answer if he/she has or does not have a nonstigmatizing characteristic. In other cases, such as the technique of Tian et al. (2007) a respondent provides a response about his/her status as related to the sensitive characteristic and a nonsensitive one, in such a way that the response provided is not enough to infer whether he/she belongs to the sensitive group. Details of the non randomized models will be presented in Chap. 6.

3.7 Surveys with Negative Questions

Assuming that in a survey questionnaire where a question has k possible answers, let only one be applicable to each participant. If the question is of sensitive nature, obviously, directly, and truthfully responding to it may jeopardize one's privacy. Following Esponda (2006) let us call such a survey, "a positive question survey." Such a survey of course is a direct response survey which exhibits all the pathology that indirect questioning techniques are trying to remedy. In contrast, assume that we have a questionnaire in which a question has k possible answers and the participant is asked to disclose one of the possible choices which does apply to him/her. Observe that the possible choices in a positive questionnaire are exhaustive and mutually exclusive in such a way that only one possible answer is applicable. In a negative questionnaire, one and only one possible answer should be false. As a result, a participant's response in a negative survey is expected to provide less information about one's status related to a sensitive characteristic. It is clear that with the use of a negative questionnaire the privacy of participants is protected and at the same time a respondent feels comfortable that by providing an option which does not apply to him/her rather than the option applicable, his/her privacy is not in jeopardy. We will discuss this technique in more detail in Chap. 6. Surveys with negative questions are expected to increase the perceived protection of privacy, i.e., the protection as it is subjectively understood by a participant. This important notion of perceived protection of privacy will be explained in Chap. 7.

References

Chaudhuri, A. (2001a). Using randomized response from a complex survey to estimate a sensitive proportion in a dichotomous finite population. *Journal of Statistical Planning and Inference*, *94*, 37–42.

Chaudhuri, A. (2001b). Estimating sensitive proportions from unequal probability samples using randomized responses. *Pakistan Journal of Statistics*, *17*, 259–270.

Chaudhuri, A. (2010). *Essentials of survey sampling*. New Delhi: Prentice Hall of India.

Chaudhuri, A. (2011). *Randomized response and indirect questioning techniques in surveys*. Boca Raton: Chapman & Hall, CRC Press, Taylor & Francis Group.

Chaudhuri, A., & Christofides, T.C. (2008). Indirect questioning: how to rival randomized response techniques. *International Journal of Pure and Applied Mathematics*, *43*, 283–294.

Christofides, T.C. (2009). Randomized response without a randomization device. *Advances and Applications in Statistics*, *11*, 15–28.

Droitcour, J.A., Larson, E.M., Scheuren, F.J. (2001). The three card method: estimating sensitive items with permanent anonymity of response. In *Proceedings of the Social Statistics Section of the American Statistical Association*. Alexandria, VA: ASA.

References

Esponda, F. (2006). Negative surveys. arXiv:ST/0608176v1

Esponda, F., & Guerrero, V.M. (2009). Surveys with negative questions for sensitive items. *Statistics and Probability Letters, 79*, 2456–2461.

Miller, J.D. (1985). The nominative technique: a new method of estimating heroin prevalence. *NIDA Research Monograph*, (57), 104–124.

Miller, J.D., Cisin, I.H., Harrel, A.V. (1986). A new technique for surveying deviant behavior: item count estimates of marijuana, cocaine and heroin. *Paper presented at the annual meeting of the American Association for Public Opinion Research*, St. Petersburg, Florida.

Tan, M.T., Tian, G.L., Tang, M.L. (2009). Sample surveys with sensitive questions: a non-randomized response approach. *American Statistician, 63*, 9–16.

Tian, G.-L., Yu, J.-W., Tang, M.-L., Geng, Z. (2007). A new nonrandomized model for analyzing sensitive questions with binary outcomes. *Statistics in Medicine, 26*, 4238–4252.

Warner, S.L. (1965). Randomized Response: a survey technique for eliminating evasive answer bias. *Journal of the American Statistical Association, 60*, 63–69.

Yu, J.-W., Tian, G.-L., Tang, M.-L. (2008). Two new models for survey sampling with sensitive characteristic: design and analysis. *Metrika, 67*, 251–263.

Chapter 4
Randomized Response Techniques to Capture Qualitative Features

Abstract This chapter is devoted entirely to randomized response techniques which can be implemented to estimate certain parameters of a qualitative stigmatizing characteristic. Descriptions of the randomized response procedures of specific techniques are given. In particular details are provided for Warner's, Simmon's, Kuk's, Christofides', and the Forced Response randomized response techniques. For those techniques, explicit formulae are given for the various estimators of interest and measures of their accuracy, assuming that the sample is chosen according to a general sampling design. However, given that most practitioners are more familiar with simple random sampling without replacement, the formulae are explicitly stated for this particular sampling scheme as well. In addition to the numerous randomized response techniques reviewed, this chapter includes a recently developed randomized response technique which uses the Poisson distribution to estimate parameters related to a stigmatizing characteristic which is extremely rare. Furthermore, we discuss an approach using the geometric distribution to generate randomized responses. Also in this chapter, techniques dealing with multiple sensitive characteristics are described. Finally, some aspects of the Bayesian approach in analyzing randomized response data are presented along with a brief literature review on the topic.

4.1 Introduction

We restrict to a finite survey population $U = (1, \ldots, i, \ldots, N)$ of a known number N of identifiable persons labeled $i = 1, \ldots, N$. The member i of the population bears a value y_i of a variable y defined on U. Each y_i assumes either one of the two real values 0 or 1. If $y_i = 1$, the person bears a stigmatizing qualitative feature A; if $y_i = 0$, the person bears the complementary characteristic A^c. For example, A may mean alcoholism, implying A^c is innocuous. If A means supportive of a particular political party, then in certain societies A^c may also be a sensitive feature. Thus A is sensitive but A^c may be either innocuous or sensitive. Suitable randomized response techniques are to be adopted to gather truthful data from sampled persons protecting individual privacy in reasonable manners. Few such devices will be briefly described with an intention to estimate $\theta = \left(\sum_{i=1}^{N} y_i\right)/N$ which is the proportion bearing the sensitive feature A in the community of N people. Properties of the proposed estimators will be discussed.

On hitting upon an appropriate sampling design p, a sample s of a suitable number of units n, $(n < N)$ from U has to be first selected and surveyed for the values y_i for all i in s. Then, an appropriate estimator for θ will have to be hit upon involving the units in s and the respective values for them as gathered through a randomized response device employed and executed.

We shall illustrate specific randomized response devices in the next section but here in a general way we discuss general estimation procedures.

For every sampled person i in s by a randomized response device we shall elicit suitably a response, say, r_i independently across the various separate persons. Denoting generically the expectation operators over the design p by E_p and over the randomization response device by E_R, the variance operators correspondingly by V_p, V_R, the covariance operator over the randomized response technique by C_R, and by E and V the overall expectation and variance operator, respectively, we shall presume the following:

$$E = E_p E_R = E_R E_p$$

and

$$V = E_p V_R + V_p E_R = E_R V_p + V_R E_p$$

i.e., the operators are commutative. The design p will be so selected that

$$\pi_i = \sum_{s \ni i} p(s) > 0, \ \forall \ i \in U$$

and

$$\pi_{ij} = \sum_{s \ni i,j} p(s) > 0, \forall \ i, j \in U, i \neq j.$$

These are, respectively, the inclusion probabilities of the first two orders for the units i and the paired units i, j $(i \neq j)$ in U; π_{ii} of course is π_i itself.

For $Y = \sum_{i=1}^{N} y_i$ we shall usually employ the estimator $e = \sum_{i \in s} (r_i/\pi_i)$ and the estimator e/N for $\theta = Y/N$. The randomized response device is so employed that

$$E_R(r_i) = y_i,$$
$$V_R(r_i) = \alpha + \beta y_i = V_i,$$

say, with α, β known. Consequently, $v_i = \alpha + \beta r_i$ has

$$E_R(v_i) = V_i,$$

$$E(e) = E_P\left(\sum_{i \in s} \frac{y_i}{\pi_i}\right) = Y = E_R\left(\sum_{i=1}^N r_i\right),$$

$$V(e) = E_P\left(\sum_{i \in s} \frac{V_i}{\pi_i^2}\right) + V_P\left(\sum_{i \in s} \frac{y_i}{\pi_i}\right)$$

$$= \sum_{i=1}^N \frac{V_i}{\pi_i} + \sum_i \sum_{j,j>i} (\pi_i \pi_j - \pi_{ij})\left(\frac{y_i}{\pi_i} - \frac{y_j}{\pi_j}\right)^2$$

because for $t = \sum_{i \in s}(y_i/\pi_i)$, the above-noted variance formula given by Yates and Grundy (1953) is applicable, on our assumption that every sample has a fixed number of units in it that are all distinct.

A design unbiased estimator for $V_p(t)$ due to Yates and Grundy (1953) is

$$v_p(t) = \sum_{i \in s} \sum_{j \in s, j > i} \left(\frac{\pi_i \pi_j - \pi_{ij}}{\pi_{ij}}\right)\left(\frac{y_i}{\pi_i} - \frac{y_j}{\pi_j}\right)^2.$$

Then, an unbiased estimator of $V(e)$ is

$$v(e) = v_p(t)\,|_{\underline{Y}=\underline{R}} + \sum_{i \in s} \frac{v_i}{\pi_i}.$$

Here $\underline{Y} = (y_1, \ldots, y_i, \ldots, y_N)$, $\underline{R} = (r_1, \ldots, r_i, \ldots, r_N)$, and $v_p(t)\,|_{\underline{Y}=\underline{R}}$ stands for $v_p(t)$ evaluated at $\underline{Y}$ taken at $\underline{R}$.

Later, when needed, we shall consider specific sampling designs and schemes, specific alternative forms of t, $V_p(t)$, e, $V(e)$, $v_p(t)$, and $v(e)$.

Next follows description of specific randomized response devices.

4.2 Warner's, Simmons's, Kuk's, Forced Response, and Christofides's RRT

We shall write $y_i = 1$ if i bears A and $y_i = 0$ if i bears A^c. Warner's (1965) randomized response device works as follows. A sampled person labeled i is offered a box of a considerable number of identical cards with a proportion p $(0 < p < 1$, $p \neq 0.5)$ of them marked A and the rest marked A^c. The person is requested, outside of view of the interviewer, to shuffle the cards in the box, randomly draw one of them, check the card's mark, give the response I_i which is 1 if the card type "matches" his/her actual feature A or A^c and is 0 otherwise, i.e., a "mis-match" and then return the card to the box. During this process the respondent must not reveal the outcome of the experiment to the enquirer. In this Warner randomized response device it seems implied that admission of bearing A is disliked by a respondent but not admission of bearing of A^c. The response $I_i = 1$ is operationally equivalent to saying "Yes" and $I_i = 0$ is equivalent to saying "No." Directly saying "Yes" about A or "No" about A^c is clearly feared to be "revealing" an undesired "trait" and hence disliked by a respondent. But since the card type found is kept a secret, an answer "Yes" or "No" about it is supposed to be unrevealing of the feature A borne by the sampled person. Using the "Yes" and "No" responses from a "simple random sample" taken "with replacement" Warner (1965) found it easy to

- estimate $\theta = \frac{1}{N} \sum_{i=1}^{N} y_i$,
- obtain the variance of the estimate, and
- to unbiasedly estimate this variance.

We shall not report the details here but postpone to the next Sect. 4.3. Horvitz, Shah, and Simmons (1967) and Greenberg, Abul-Ela, Simmons, and Horvitz (1969) have narrated an alternative randomized response device invented by Simmons with the same purpose to suitably estimate θ from a sample of respondents, presumably supposing both A and A^c sensitive enough so that a person is unlikely to directly say "Yes" or "No" about bearing either A or A^c. In the randomized response device proposed by Simmons, besides the stigmatizing attribute, an innocuous attribute B is visualized which is admittedly unrelated to A. For example, a person preferring music to sports may be supposed to bear the innocuous characteristic B. His/her attribute will be B^c if the preference is for sports to music. Either feature B or B^c need not influence a person to bear the characteristic A of being, say, a habitual tax evader, i.e., the innocuous and sensitive characteristics are independent. First the proportion θ_B of people bearing B is supposed to be known. Introducing a variable x and writing its value x_i for a person labeled i, one may take $\theta_B = \left(\sum_{i=1}^{N} x_i \right)/N$ because one may define $x_i = 1$ if i bears B and $x_i = 0$ if i bears the complementary trait B^c.

The randomized response device of Simmons then presents to a sampled person labeled i a box with a large number of identical cards with a proportion p ($0 < p < 1$) bearing the mark A and the rest marked B. The response solicited denoted by I_i takes the value 1 if i bears A and the card drawn is marked A or if i bears B and the card drawn is marked B. Otherwise I_i takes on the value 0. Observe that $I_i = 1$ is equivalent to a "Yes" response while $I_i = 0$ represents the case of a "No" response. In case θ_B is known, Horvitz et al. (1967) and Greenberg et al. (1969) above give an estimator for θ, the variance of this estimator and an estimator thereof using these randomized responses based on a simple random sample with replacement taken in n draws. But if θ_B is not known, which is a more realistic situation, two independent simple random samples with replacement in n_1 draws and n_2 draws in the first and second are taken. Moreover, in the first sample a

4.2 Warner's, Simmons's, Kuk's, Forced Response, and Christofides's RRT

box of cards with a proportion p_1 ($0 < p_1 < 1$) bearing A and in the second the corresponding proportion p as p_2 ($0 < p_2 < 1$) are taken. Obviously the outcomes of drawing the cards from the boxes are not to be disclosed by the respondents to the enquirers. Estimation of θ, derivation of the variance, and estimation of the latter are easily accomplished. Chaudhuri (2001a,b, 2010) slightly revised this Simmons randomized response device by requiring only a single sample but two independent randomized responses from each sampled person using two boxes with identical cards marked A, B in proportions $p_1 : (1 - p_1)$ in the first and $p_2 : (1 - p_2)$ in the second box, respectively. Detailed estimation procedure is related in Sect. 4.3.

Kuk (1990) generalized Warner's (1965) randomized response device essentially in the following way which is being narrated as Chaudhuri's (2010, 2011) version of the latter. A sampled person i is offered two boxes. Each box contains identical cards of two colors only, red and white, in sufficiently large numbers with proportions $p_1 : (1 - p_1)$ in the first and $p_2 : (1 - p_2)$ in the second. A person sampled is requested to use the first box, if his/her trait is A and the second box if his/her trait is A^c and to make K independent draws of cards with replacement each. The person reports f_i, which is the number of times a red card is drawn. In Sect. 4.3, detailed estimation procedures are described.

The "Forced Response" randomized response technique was introduced by Boruch (1972) as elaborately discussed further by Fox and Tracy (1986), Chaudhuri and Mukerjee (1988), and Chaudhuri (2011) among others. To apply this, a sampled person i is offered a box containing a number of identical cards with a proportion p_1 ($0 < p_1 < 1$) of them marked A, a proportion p_2 ($0 < p_2 < 1$) marked A^c and the remaining proportion $p_3 = 1 - p_1 - p_2$ ($0 < p_1 + p_2 < 1$) of the cards "unmarked" or marked blank. The sampled person i is to report I_i which is as follows:

$I_i = 1$ if the card type A or A^c matches the person's trait or if a blank card comes up and the person bears A

or

$I_i = 0$ if the card type A or A^c mismatches his/her trait or if a blank card is drawn and the person bears A^c.

The card drawn must be returned to the box after reporting the value of I_i. In Sect. 4.3 the estimation theory is presented for simple random sampling with replacement and general samples.

Christofides (2003), restricting to simple random sampling with replacement, gives the following randomized response technique. A sampled person i is given a box with identical cards bearing each a separate mark as $1, \ldots, k, \ldots, M$ with $M \geq 2$ but in known proportions $p_1, \ldots, p_k, \ldots, p_M$ with $0 < p_k < 1$ for $k = 1, \ldots, M$ and $\sum_{k=1}^{M} p_k = 1$. The person sampled is requested to draw one of the cards and respond

- k if a card marked k is drawn and the person bears A^c or
- $M - k + 1$ if a card marked k is drawn but the person bears A.

After responding, the card is to be returned to the box. Chaudhuri (2004) extended this to cover a sample chosen by a general scheme. The theory of estimation is presented elaborately in Sect. 4.3.

4.3 Related Estimation in SRSWR and Sophisticated Sampling

The reading of a description of a randomized response technique in a publication gives often an impression that it is inalienably linked with a specific method about how a sample has been chosen. But as emphasized in the recent monograph of Chaudhuri (2011), given any sampled person, no matter how selected, any specific randomized response device may be freely employed and that too in independent manners.

A second important issue we intend to thrash out is that a theory of estimation based on a linear estimator in Godambe's (1955) sense involving real values y_i for i in a sample s chosen according to a design is first assumed to be developed. Replacing each y_i by a suitable randomized response based unbiased estimator for it, the theory for direct response data is to be revised to provide one for randomized response data.

In analogy with a theory of multi-stage sampling, randomized response theory involves a loss in precision compared to an underlying direct response theory on which the former is only an adjustment.

Let $\underline{Y} = (y_1, \ldots, y_i, \ldots, y_N)$, Y_k be the value of y for a unit chosen on the k-th draw in a sample taken in a simple random sampling with replacement in n draws. For a direct response survey an unbiased estimator for

$$\bar{Y} = \frac{1}{N} \sum_{i=1}^{N} y_i = \theta,$$

the proportion of people bearing A in $U = (1, \ldots, i, \ldots, N)$ is the sample mean

$$\bar{y} = \frac{1}{n} \sum_{k=1}^{n} Y_k = \hat{\theta},$$

say. Then,

$$V(\bar{y}) = \frac{\sigma^2}{n}, \quad \sigma^2 = \frac{1}{N} \sum_{i=1}^{N} (y_i - \bar{Y})^2.$$

4.3 Related Estimation in SRSWR and Sophisticated Sampling

Writing

$$s^2 = \frac{1}{n-1} \sum_{k=1}^{n} (Y_k - \bar{y})^2,$$

an unbiased estimator for $V(\hat{y})$ is

$$\frac{s^2}{n} = v(\bar{y}).$$

Noting that each y_i is either 1 or 0, one gets

$$V(\bar{y}) = \frac{\theta(1-\theta)}{n}, \quad v(\bar{y}) = \frac{\hat{\theta}(1-\hat{\theta})}{n-1}.$$

For Warner's (1965) randomized response device, let

$$I_k = \begin{cases} 1 & \text{if the person chosen on the } k\text{-th draw finds a "match" in card type and trait} \\ 0 & \text{if a "no-match" is encountered.} \end{cases}$$

Then,

$$E_R(I_k) = (1-p) + (2p-1)y_k$$

and

$$r_k = \frac{I_k - (1-p)}{2p-1}$$

has

$$E_R(r_k) = y_k \text{ and } V_R(I_k) = \frac{p(1-p)}{(2p-1)^2}.$$

In addition,

$$\bar{r} = \frac{1}{n} \sum_{k=1}^{n} r_k$$

with $\underline{R} = (r_1, \ldots, r_i, \ldots, r_N)$ has $E(\bar{r}) = E_p(\bar{y}) = \bar{Y}$ (since $E_R(\bar{r}) = \bar{y}$),

$$V(\bar{r}) = V(\bar{y}) + \frac{p(1-p)}{n(2p-1)^2} = \frac{1}{n}\left[\theta(1-\theta) + \frac{p(1-p)}{(2p-1)^2}\right].$$

and

$$v(\bar{r}) = \frac{1}{n-1}\left[\hat{\theta}(1-\hat{\theta}) + \frac{p(1-p)}{(2p-1)^2}\right]$$

is an unbiased estimator of $V(\bar{y})$ while $\bar{r}$ is an unbiased estimator for θ.

Clearly, the value chosen for p is important in the quantifications of $\bar{r}$ and both $V(\bar{r})$ and $v(\bar{r})$. A value of p chosen close to 0.5 will induce in a respondent a greater faith in the procedure in protecting his/her privacy. But the closer the value of p to 0.5, the higher the magnitudes of $v(\bar{r})$ and of the coefficient of variation of $\bar{r}$ namely, $CV = 100\sqrt{v(\bar{r})}/\bar{r}$. So, an intelligent balancing is needed in the choice of p, that is, the proportion of cards marked A in the box.

Assume that a sample s is chosen according to a general design p with probabilities of inclusion

$$\pi_i = \sum_{s \ni i} p(s) > 0 \text{ for } i \in U,$$

and

$$\pi_{ij} = \sum_{s \ni i,j} p(s) > 0 \text{ for } i, j \in U(i \neq j).$$

Then, for a direct response survey

$$t = \frac{1}{N}\sum_{i \in s}\frac{y_i}{\pi_i},$$

equal to $\bar{y} = \left(\sum_{i \in s} y_i\right)/n$ for simple random sampling without replacement (SRSWOR), may be used to unbiasedly estimate θ. Its variance is

$$V_p(t) = \sum_i \sum_{j,j>i}(\pi_i\pi_j - \pi_{ij})\left(\frac{y_i}{\pi_i} - \frac{y_j}{\pi_j}\right)^2$$

which in case of SRSWOR is equal to

$$\frac{N-n}{nN}S^2 \text{ where } S^2 = \frac{1}{N-1}\sum_{i=1}^{N}(y_i - \bar{Y})^2,$$

assuming each sample contains a fixed number of units, each distinct. An unbiased estimator for it is

$$v_p(t) = \sum_{i \in s}\sum_{j \in s, j>i}\left(\frac{\pi_i\pi_j - \pi_{ij}}{\pi_{ij}}\right)\left(\frac{y_i}{\pi_i} - \frac{y_j}{\pi_j}\right)^2,$$

4.3 Related Estimation in SRSWR and Sophisticated Sampling

which, for SRSWOR is equal to

$$\frac{N-n}{nN}s^2 \text{ where } s^2 = \frac{1}{n-1}\sum_{i \in s}(y_i - \bar{y})^2.$$

In case randomized response data are only available, then we shall write

$$I_i = \begin{cases} 1 & \text{if card type "matches" the trait of the person labeled } i, A \text{ or } A^c \\ 0 & \text{if a "non-match" results.} \end{cases}$$

Then, for Warner's randomized response device

$$r_i = \frac{I_i - (1-p)}{2p-1}, \ p \neq \frac{1}{2}$$

will unbiasedly estimate y_i, $i \in U$. Also,

$$e = \frac{1}{N}\sum_{i \in s}\frac{r_i}{\pi_i} \text{ equal to } \bar{r} = \frac{1}{n}\sum_{i \in s}r_i$$

for SRSWOR, will have

$$E_P(e) = \frac{1}{N}\sum_{i=1}^{N}r_i = \frac{R}{N} = \bar{R}$$

$$E_R(e) = \frac{1}{N}\sum_{i \in s}\frac{y_i}{\pi_i} = t$$

and hence

$$E(e) = E_R[E_P(e)] = E_P[E_R(e)] = \theta.$$

Also

$$V_R(r_i) = \frac{p(1-p)}{(2p-1)^2} = V_i, \forall i \in U,$$

$$V_R(e) = \frac{1}{N^2}\sum_{i \in s}\frac{V_i}{\pi_i^2} = \frac{p(1-p)}{(2p-1)^2}\frac{1}{N^2}\sum_{i \in s}\frac{1}{\pi_i^2}$$

$$V_P(e) = \frac{1}{N^2}\sum_{i}\sum_{j,j>i}(\pi_i\pi_j - \pi_{ij})\left(\frac{r_i}{\pi_i} - \frac{r_j}{\pi_j}\right)^2,$$

which is equal to

$$\frac{N-n}{nN(N-1)} \sum_{i=1}^{N} (r_i - \bar{R})^2$$

for SRSWOR,

$$v_p(e) = \frac{1}{N^2} \sum_{i} \sum_{j,j>i} \left(\frac{\pi_i \pi_j - \pi_{ij}}{\pi_{ij}} \right) \left(\frac{r_i}{\pi_i} - \frac{r_j}{\pi_j} \right)^2,$$

equal to

$$\frac{N-n}{nN(n-1)} \sum_{i \in s} (r_i - \bar{r})^2$$

for SRSWOR. So,

$$V(e) = E_p V_R(e) + V_p E_R(e)$$

$$= \frac{1}{N^2} \left[\frac{p(1-p)}{(2p-1)^2} \sum_{i=1}^{N} \frac{1}{\pi_i} + \sum_{i} \sum_{j,j>i} (\pi_i \pi_j - \pi_{ij}) \left(\frac{y_i}{\pi_i} - \frac{y_j}{\pi_j} \right)^2 \right]$$

$$= E_R V_p(e) + V_R E_p(e)$$

$$= \frac{1}{N^2} \left[\sum_{i} \sum_{j,j>i} (\pi_i \pi_j - \pi_{ij}) E_R \left(\frac{r_i}{\pi_i} - \frac{r_j}{\pi_j} \right)^2 + \frac{Np(1-p)}{(2p-1)^2} \right],$$

equal to

$$\frac{N-n}{nN(N-1)} \sum_{i=1}^{N} (y_i - \bar{Y})^2 + \frac{p(1-p)}{N(2p-1)^2},$$

for SRSWOR. Thus, an unbiased estimator for $V(e)$ is

$$v(e) = \frac{1}{N^2} \left[\sum_{i \in s} \sum_{j \in s, j > i} \left(\frac{\pi_i \pi_j - \pi_{ij}}{\pi_{ij}} \right) \left(\frac{r_i}{\pi_i} - \frac{r_j}{\pi_j} \right)^2 + \frac{p(1-p)}{(2p-1)^2} \sum_{i \in s} \frac{1}{\pi_i} \right],$$

equal to

$$\frac{N-n}{nN(n-1)} \sum_{i \in s} (r_i - \bar{r})^2 + \frac{p(1-p)}{n(2p-1)^2}$$

for SRSWOR.

4.3 Related Estimation in SRSWR and Sophisticated Sampling

In order to emphasize how one should be guided in hitting upon an appropriate "strategy," namely "A combination of a sampling design and an estimator for θ to be based on a sample drawn according to such a design" let us proceed as follows.

One particularly useful and simple such strategy is given by Rao, Hartley, and Cochran (1962). In this, choosing a sample size n ($n < N$), the population U is divided into n random groups. The i-th group is composed of N_i units taken by Simple Random Sampling Without Replacement (SRSWOR) method starting with $i = 1$ and then successively from U of N units, $N - N_1$, $N - N_1 - N_2$, units and so on with N_n units from $N - N_1 - \cdots - N_{n-1}$ units of U; The N_i's are suitably chosen with $\sum_n N_i = N$ where $\sum_n$ denotes the sum over the n random groups. The units of U are supposed to have known positive-valued size-measures $X_1, X_2, \ldots, X_N$ such that $X = \sum_i X_i$. Let $P_i = X_i/X$, $i \in U$. These P_i-values are called the normed size-measures. For the N_i units $i_1, \ldots, i_j, \ldots i_{Ni}$ falling in the i-th random group, let these P_i-values be $P_{i1}, \ldots, P_{iNi}$ and let

$$Q_i = P_{i1} + \cdots + P_{iNi}, \ i = 1, \ldots, n.$$

Then, $\sum_{i=1}^{n} Q_i = 1$. Now from the i-th group just one unit, say, i_j is to be selected with probability P_{ij}/Q_i and this step is to be independently repeated for each of the n random groups already formed. Then,

$$t_{RHC} = \sum_n y_{ij} \left(\frac{Q_i}{P_{ij}}\right)$$

is an unbiased estimator for Y, called the Rao–Hartley–Cochran estimator. Its variance is

$$V_p(t_{RHC}) = C \sum_i \sum_{i', i' > i} P_i P_{i'} \left(\frac{y_i}{P_i} - \frac{y_{i'}}{P_{i'}}\right)^2,$$

writing for simplicity y_i, P_i as the y-value and P-value for the unit chosen form the i-th group and $C = \left(\sum_n N_i^2 - N\right) / (N(N-1))$. An unbiased estimator for this variance is

$$v_p(t_{RHC}) = D \sum_n \sum_{n'} Q_i Q_{i'} \left(\frac{y_i}{P_i} - \frac{y_{i'}}{P_{i'}}\right)^2$$

where $D = \left(\sum_n N_i^2 - N\right) / \left(N^2 - \sum_n N_i^2\right)$; $\sum_n \sum_{n'}$ denotes sum over the distinct pairs of groups with no repetition.

When instead of direct response data, only randomized response data are gathered as r_i for i in s independently across these i's, then the Rao, Hartley, and Cochran strategy will be revised employing the unbiased estimator for Y which is

$$e_{RHC} = \sum_n r_i \frac{Q_i}{P_i},$$

(and of course e_{RHC}/N for θ). Then its variance will be

$$V(e_{RHC}) = C \sum_i \sum_{i',i'>i} P_i P_{i'} \left(\frac{y_i}{P_i} - \frac{y_{i'}}{P_{i'}}\right)^2 + \sum_i V_i \left(\frac{1}{P_i} - 1\right),$$

of course with $V_i = V_R(r_i), i \in U$. An unbiased estimator for $V(e_{RHC})$ is

$$v(e_{RHC}) = D \sum_n \sum_{n'} Q_i Q_{i'} \left(\frac{r_i}{P_i} - \frac{r_{i'}}{P_{j'}}\right)^2 + \sum_n V_i \frac{Q_i}{P_i};$$

this is because $V_i = p(1-p)/(2p-1)^2$ is known for the Warner (1965) randomized response device. For other randomized response devices we shall presently note that in unbiased variance estimator formulae, V_i will be replaced by an estimator for it, namely v_i such that $E_R(v_i) = V_i$.

In the context of direct response surveys, a rich literature exists to guide us in choosing among competing strategies in terms of the magnitudes of $V_p(t)$ for various combinations (p, t). Assessment from a sample is carried out in terms of the estimated coefficient of variation as $CV = 100\sqrt{v_p(t)}/t$. But in judging among (p, e) we have to evaluate $V(e)$ which involves V_i and the b_{si}'s involved in the choice

$$t = \sum_{i \in s} = y_i b_{si} \text{ and } e = \sum_{i \in s} r_i b_{si}$$

with b_{si} free of $\underline{Y} = (y_1, \ldots, y_i, \ldots, y_N)$ and $\underline{R} = (r_1, \ldots, r_i, \ldots, r_N)$ subject to

$$\sum_{s \ni i} p(s) b_{si} = 1 \text{ for all } i \in U.$$

Assessment after the sample is drawn and surveyed will be again in terms of the coefficient of variation $CV = 100\sqrt{v(e)}/e$, which will involve V_i or its estimator v_i, if V_i is not known.

For the Unrelated Question Model of Simmons let us consider the above estimation aspects. Let the first box with cards marked be in proportions $p_1 : (1 - p_1)$ and the second box in proportions $p_2 : (1 - p_2)$, $p_1 \neq p_2$. Let

$$I_i = \begin{cases} 1 & \text{if card type drawn ``matches'' the sensitive trait } A \text{ or the innocuous trait } B \\ 0 & \text{if there is ``non-match'' with the first box.} \end{cases}$$

and let

4.3 Related Estimation in SRSWR and Sophisticated Sampling

$$J_i = \begin{cases} 1 & \text{if there is "match" for the second box} \\ 0 & \text{if there is "non-match" for the second box.} \end{cases}$$

Let us recall

$$y_i = \begin{cases} 1 & \text{if } i \text{ bears } A \\ 0 & \text{if } i \text{ bears } A^c \end{cases}$$

and

$$x_i = \begin{cases} 1 & \text{if } i \text{ bears } B \\ 0 & \text{if } i \text{ bears } B^c. \end{cases}$$

Then,

$$E_R(I_i) = p_1 y_i + (1 - p_1) x_i,$$
$$E_R(J_i) = p_2 y_i + (1 - p_2) x_i$$

and

$$r_i = \frac{(1 - p_2) I_i - (1 - p_1) J_i}{p_1 - p_2}, \quad i \in U,$$

$$E_R(r_i) = y_i,$$

$$V_R(I_i) = E_R(I_i) [1 - E_R(I_i)],$$

$$V_R(J_i) = E_R(J_i) [1 - E_R(J_i)],$$

$$V_R(r_i) = \frac{(1 - p_2)^2 V_R(I_i) + (1 - p_1)^2 V_R(J_i)}{(p_1 - p_2)^2} = V_i.$$

Since

$$V_R(r_i) = E_R(r_i^2) - (E_R(r_i))^2$$
$$= E_R(r_i^2) - y_i^2$$
$$= E_R(r_i^2) - y_i$$
$$= E_R(r_i^2 - r_i)$$
$$= E_R[r_i(r_i - 1)],$$

then $v_i = r_i(r_i - 1)$ provides an unbiased estimator for

$$V_i = \frac{(1-p_1)(1-p_2)(p_1+p_2-2p_1p_2)}{(p_1-p_2)^2}(y_i - x_i)^2. \tag{4.1}$$

The next steps under this unrelated question model will be quite analogous to those noted for the Warner (1965) model. If a sample is taken by simple random sampling with replacement, then in this case also we shall write r_k to denote the r_i-value for the person chosen on the k-th draw, $k = 1, \ldots, n$. For $\theta = \left(\sum_{i=1}^{N} y_i\right)/N$ an unbiased estimator will be taken as

$$\bar{r} = \frac{1}{n}\sum_{k=1}^{n} r_k = \hat{\theta},$$

say. Then

$$V(\bar{r}) = \frac{1}{n}\left[\theta(1-\theta) + \frac{1}{N}\sum_{i=1}^{N} V_i\right]$$

with V_i as in (4.1). An unbiased estimator for this $V(\bar{r})$ is

$$v(\bar{r}) = \frac{1}{n-1}\left[\hat{\theta}(1-\hat{\theta}) + \frac{1}{n}\sum_{k=1}^{n} r_k(r_k - 1)\right].$$

For an arbitrary design with positive-valued π_i and π_{ij}, the version of the Horvitz and Thompson's (1952) estimator for θ is

$$e = \frac{1}{N}\sum_{i \in s} \frac{r_i}{\pi_i},$$

equal to $\bar{r} = \left(\sum_{i \in s} r_i\right)/n$ for SRSWOR. Its variance is

$$V(e) = \frac{1}{N^2}\left[\sum_i \sum_{j,j>i}(\pi_i\pi_j - \pi_{ij})\left(\frac{y_i}{\pi_i} - \frac{y_j}{\pi_j}\right)^2 + \sum_{i \in s}\frac{V_i}{\pi_i}\right],$$

which is equal to

$$\frac{N-n}{nN}S^2 + \frac{1}{nN}\sum_{i \in s} V_i$$

for SRSWOR and the Yates and Grundy's (1953) unbiased estimator for this $V(e)$ is

4.3 Related Estimation in SRSWR and Sophisticated Sampling

$$v(e) = \frac{1}{N^2} \left[\sum_{i \in s} \sum_{j \in s, j > i} \left(\frac{\pi_i \pi_j - \pi_{ij}}{\pi_{ij}} \right) \left(\frac{r_i}{\pi_i} - \frac{r_j}{\pi_j} \right)^2 + \sum_{i \in s} \frac{r_i(r_i - 1)}{\pi_i} \right],$$

equal to

$$\frac{N-n}{nN(n-1)} \sum_{i \in s} (r_i - \bar{r})^2 + \frac{1}{nN} \sum_{i \in s} r_i(r_i - 1)$$

for SRSWOR.

For the Rao–Hartley–Cochran scheme, the appropriate unbiased estimator for θ is

$$e_{RHC} = \frac{1}{N} \sum_n r_i \frac{Q_i}{P_i}.$$

Its variance is

$$V(e_{RHC}) = \frac{1}{N^2} \left[C \sum_i \sum_{i', i' > i} P_i P_{i'} \left(\frac{y_i}{P_i} - \frac{y_{i'}}{P_{i'}} \right)^2 + \sum_i V_i \left(\frac{1}{P_i} - 1 \right) \right]$$

and an unbiased estimator for its variance is

$$v(e_{RHC}) = \frac{1}{N^2} \left[D \sum_n \sum_{n'} Q_i Q_{i'} \left(\frac{r_i}{P_i} - \frac{r_{i'}}{P_{i'}} \right)^2 + \sum_n r_i(r_i - 1) \frac{Q_i}{P_i} \right].$$

For Kuk's (1990) randomized response device a person sampled is offered two boxes; if the person bears A he/she is to report the number of times a red card comes up in K draws at random with replacement from the first box, with θ_1 as the proportion of the red cards in it; if the person bears A^c, this report will be similarly made using the second box with θ_2 ($\theta_2 \neq \theta_1$) as the proportion of red cards in it. First, let the sample be taken in n draws by simple random sampling with replacement. Let $f(k)$ be the response from a person chosen on the k-th draw, $k = 1, \ldots, n$. Then,

$$E_R(f(k)) = K[\theta \theta_1 + (1-\theta)\theta_2], \ \forall \ k = 1, \ldots, n,$$

and

$$V_R(f(k)) = K[\theta \theta_1(1-\theta_1) + (1-\theta)\theta_2(1-\theta_2)]$$
$$= K[\theta_2(1-\theta_2) + \theta(\theta_1 - \theta_2)(1 - \theta_1 - \theta_2)].$$

Let

$$r(k) = \frac{1}{\theta_1 - \theta_2} \left[\frac{f(k)}{K} - \theta_2 \right]$$

so that $E_R(r(k)) = \theta$ for every $k = 1, \ldots, n$. Consequently,

$$\bar{r} = \frac{1}{n} \sum_{k=1}^{n} r(k)$$

has $E(\bar{r}) = \theta$, i.e., $\bar{r}$ is Kuk's unbiased estimator for θ. Then

$$V(\bar{r}) = V_p(\bar{y}) + E_p \left[\frac{V_R(f(k))}{nK(\theta_1 - \theta_2)^2} \right]$$

$$= \frac{\theta(1-\theta)}{n} + \frac{\alpha + \beta\theta}{n},$$

where

$$\alpha = \frac{\theta_2(1-\theta_2)}{K(\theta_1 - \theta_2)^2}, \quad \beta = \frac{1 - \theta_1 - \theta_2}{K(\theta_1 - \theta_2)}.$$

Then,

$$v(\bar{r}) = \frac{\bar{r}(1-\bar{r})}{n-1} + \frac{1}{n}(\alpha + \beta\bar{r})$$

is an unbiased estimator of $V(\bar{r})$.

For a general sampling design with positive-valued inclusion probabilities π_i for a person i and π_{ij} that for a pair of distinct persons i and j, $(i \neq j)$ in $U = (1, \ldots, i, \ldots, N)$ with randomized response data gathered through Kuk's device, we should proceed as follows.

For a person labeled i the randomized response is f_i, the number of red cards drawn. Then,

$$E_R(f_i) = K[\theta_1 y_i + \theta_2 (1 - y_i)]$$

giving

$$r_i = \left(\frac{f_i}{K} - \theta_2 \right) / (\theta_1 - \theta_2)$$

with $E_R(r_i) = y_i$, $i \in U$. In addition,

$$V_R(f_i) = K[\theta_1(1-\theta_1) y_i + \theta_2(1-\theta_2)(1-y_i)]$$

4.3 Related Estimation in SRSWR and Sophisticated Sampling

giving

$$V_R(r_i) = \frac{[\theta_2(1-\theta_2) + y_i(\theta_1-\theta_2)(1-\theta_1-\theta_2)]}{K(\theta_1-\theta_2)^2} = \alpha + \beta y_i = V_i$$

say, where

$$\alpha = \frac{\theta_2(1-\theta_2)}{K(\theta_1-\theta_2)^2}, \quad \beta = \frac{1-\theta_1-\theta_2}{K(\theta_1-\theta_2)}.$$

So, $v_i = \alpha + \beta r_i$ satisfies $E_R(v_i) = V_i$, $i \in U$. Then, an unbiased estimator for θ may be taken as

$$e = \frac{1}{N} \sum_{i \in s} \frac{r_i}{\pi_i}$$

equal to $\bar{r} = \left(\sum_{i \in s} r_i\right)/n$ for SRSWOR. Then, $E(e) = \theta$ with

$$V(e) = \frac{1}{N^2} \left[\sum_i \sum_{j,j>i} (\pi_i \pi_j - \pi_{ij}) \left(\frac{y_i}{\pi_i} - \frac{y_j}{\pi_j} \right)^2 + \sum_{i=1}^{N} \frac{V_i}{\pi_i} \right],$$

equal to

$$\frac{N-n}{nN(N-1)} \sum_{i=1}^{N} (y_i - \bar{Y})^2 + \frac{1}{nN} \sum_{i=1}^{N} V_i$$

for SRSWOR.
An unbiased estimator for it following Yates and Grundy (1953) is

$$v(e) = \frac{1}{N^2} \left[\sum_{i \in s} \sum_{j \in s, j>i} \left(\frac{\pi_i \pi_j - \pi_{ij}}{\pi_{ij}} \right) \left(\frac{r_i}{\pi_i} - \frac{r_j}{\pi_j} \right)^2 + \sum_{i \in s} \frac{v_i}{\pi_i} \right],$$

equal to

$$\frac{N-n}{nN(n-1)} \sum_{i \in s} (r_i - \bar{r})^2 + \frac{1}{nN} \sum_{i \in s} v_i$$

for SRSWOR.

If the Rao et al. (1962) scheme is adopted in sampling, then, with r_i, V_i and v_i given as earlier, θ may be unbiasedly estimated by

$$e_{RHC} = \frac{1}{N} \sum_n r_i \frac{Q_i}{P_i}$$

having of course $E(e_{RHC}) = 0$. In addition,

$$V(e_{RHC}) = \frac{1}{N^2}\left[C\sum_i\sum_{j,j>i}P_iP_j\left(\frac{y_i}{P_i}-\frac{y_j}{P_j}\right)^2 + \sum_i V_i\left(\frac{1}{P_i}-1\right)\right].$$

Then

$$v(e_{RHC}) = \frac{1}{N^2}\left[D\sum_n\sum_{n'}Q_iQ_{i'}\left(\frac{r_i}{P_i}-\frac{r_{i'}}{P_{i'}}\right)^2 + \sum_n v_i\frac{Q_i}{P_i}\right]$$

is an unbiased estimator for $V(e_{RHC})$.

Next we consider the "Forced Response" randomized response device introduced by Boruch (1972) and later studied by Fox and Tracy (1986) and also dealt with by Chaudhuri and Mukerjee (1988) and Chaudhuri (2011) among others.

A sampled person labeled i is offered a box with cards marked "Yes," a few marked "No" and the rest marked genuine in respective proportions

$$p_1, p_2, 1 - p_1 - p_2, \quad (0 < p_1, p_2 < 1, \ p_1 \neq p_2, \ p_1 + p_2 < 1).$$

In case a simple random sample with replacement is taken in n draws, for the k-th person, $k = 1, \ldots, n$, let I_k be the response provided and let

$$I_k = \begin{cases} 1 & \text{if the person has to say "Yes" as per instruction or genuinely} \\ 0 & \text{if the person says "No" per instruction or because of "no match."} \end{cases}$$

Then,

$$E_R(I_k) = p_1 + (1 - p_1 - p_2)\theta = \lambda,$$

say, because θ is the common probability for any person chosen in any draw by simple random sampling with replacement if his/her trait is A. Letting

$$r_k = \frac{I_k - p_1}{1 - p_1 - p_2}$$

one gets $E_R(r_k) = \theta$. So,

$$\bar{r} = \frac{1}{n}\sum_{k=1}^n r_k$$

may be taken as an unbiased estimator for θ. Now,

$$V_R(I_k) = E_R(I_k)(1 - E_R(I_k)) = \lambda(1-\lambda).$$

4.3 Related Estimation in SRSWR and Sophisticated Sampling

Then,

$$V(\bar{r}) = \frac{\lambda(1-\lambda)}{n}.$$

Writing

$$\hat{\lambda} = p_1 + (1 - p_1 - p_2)\bar{r}$$

it follows that $E\left(\hat{\lambda}\right) = \lambda$ and hence

$$v(\bar{r}) = \frac{\hat{\lambda}(1-\hat{\lambda})}{n-1}.$$

is an unbiased estimator for $V(\bar{r})$ observing the properties of a binomial distribution as was duly observed earlier by Warner (1965).

If the sample is chosen according to a general sampling design admitting positive inclusion-probabilities π_i for i and π_{ij} for i, j ($i \neq j$) in U, then writing I_i for the response "Yes," "No" from the i-th person sampled according to this Forced Response Scheme, it follows that

$$E_R(I_i) = p_1 + (1 - p_1 - p_2) y_i$$

$$V_R(I_i) = E_R(I_i)(1 - E_R(I_i))$$
$$= p_1(1 - p_1) - (p_1 - p_2)(1 - p_1 - p_2) y_i$$

on noting $y_i^2 = y_i$ since y_i takes on the values 1 and 0. Writing

$$r_i = \frac{I_i - p_1}{1 - p_1 - p_2},$$

it follows that $E_R(r_i) = y_i$ and

$$V_R(r_i) = \frac{p_1(1 - p_1) - (p_1 - p_2)(1 - p_1 - p_2) y_i}{(1 - p_1 - p_2)^2}$$
$$= \frac{p_1(1 - p_1)}{(1 - p_1 - p_2)^2} - \frac{(p_1 - p_2) y_i}{1 - p_1 - p_2}$$
$$= \alpha + \beta y_i,$$

where

$$\alpha = \frac{p_1(1 - p_1)}{(1 - p_1 - p_2)^2}, \quad \beta = \frac{p_2 - p_1}{1 - p_1 - p_2}.$$

So,

$$e = \frac{1}{N} \sum_{i \in s} \frac{r_i}{\pi_i}$$

equal to

$$\bar{r} = \frac{1}{n} \sum_{i \in s} r_i$$

for SRSWOR, may be taken to unbiasedly estimate θ. Then,

$$V(e) = \frac{1}{N^2} \left[\sum_i \sum_{j,j>i} (\pi_i \pi_j - \pi_{ij}) \left(\frac{y_i}{\pi_i} - \frac{y_j}{\pi_j} \right)^2 + \sum_{i=1}^{N} \frac{V_i}{\pi_i} \right],$$

equal to

$$\frac{N-n}{nN} S^2 + \frac{1}{nN} \sum_{i=1}^{N} V_i$$

for SRSWOR, where $V_i = \alpha + \beta y_i$. Now taking $v_i = \alpha + \beta r_i$ so that $E_R(v_i) = V_i$, it follows that an unbiased estimator for $V(e)$ is

$$v(e) = \frac{1}{N^2} \left[\sum_{i \in s} \sum_{j \in s, j>i} \left(\frac{\pi_i \pi_j - \pi_{ij}}{\pi_{ij}} \right) \left(\frac{r_i}{\pi_i} - \frac{r_j}{\pi_j} \right)^2 + \sum \frac{v_i}{\pi_i} \right],$$

equal

$$\frac{N-n}{nN(n-1)} \sum_{i \in s} (r_i - \bar{r})^2 + \frac{1}{nN} \sum_{i \in s} v_i$$

for SRSWOR, supposing every sample contains a fixed number of units, each distinct.

If a sample s is chosen by Rao et al. (1962) scheme, then using the above notations for r_i, V_i, and v_i we may employ for θ the unbiased estimator due to Rao et al. (1962) as

$$e_{RHC} = \frac{1}{N} \sum_n r_i \frac{Q_i}{P_i}$$

with usual notations for $\sum_n$, P_i, and Q_i, $i \in U$. Then,

4.3 Related Estimation in SRSWR and Sophisticated Sampling

$$V(e_{RHC}) = \frac{1}{N^2}\left[C\sum_i\sum_{j,j>i} P_iP_j\left(\frac{y_i}{P_i} - \frac{y_j}{P_j}\right)^2 + \sum_i V_i\left(\frac{1}{P_i} - 1\right)\right]$$

and an unbiased estimator for it is

$$v(e_{RHC}) = \frac{1}{N^2}\left[D\sum_n\sum_{n'} Q_iQ_{i'}\left(\frac{r_i}{P_i} - \frac{r_{i'}}{P_{i'}}\right)^2 + \sum_n v_i\frac{Q_i}{P_i}\right].$$

Next let us consider the randomized response device given by Christofides (2003). Here a sampled person is offered a box with cards marked $1, \ldots, j, \ldots, M$ with their numbers in proportions $p_1, \ldots, p_j, \ldots, p_M$ so that

$$0 < p_j < 1, \ j = 1, \ldots, M, \ \sum_{j=1}^M p_j = 1.$$

The sampled person, on a request, is to choose one of the cards marked K, say, $K = 1, \ldots, j, \ldots, M$ and report the number K if he/she bears A^c or to report the number $M - K + 1$ if the trait is A.

If a simple random sample with replacement is chosen in n draws, then the randomized response from a person chosen on the k-th draw, $(k = 1, \ldots, n)$ is z_k, say, and

$$E_R(z_k) = \theta\left(M + 1 - \sum_{K=1}^M Kp_K\right) + (1-\theta)\sum_{K=1}^M Kp_K$$
$$= \theta(M + 1 - 2\mu) + \mu$$

where $\mu = \sum_{K=1}^M Kp_K$. So,

$$r_k = \frac{z_k - \mu}{M + 1 - 2\mu}$$

has $E_R(r_k) = \theta$ for every $k = 1, \ldots, n$ and

$$\bar{r} = \frac{1}{n}\sum_{k=1}^n r_k$$

is an unbiased estimator for θ.

Given that

$$E_R(z_k) = \theta(M + 1 - 2\mu) + \mu, \ \forall \ k = 1, \ldots, n$$

and

$$E_R(z_k^2) = \theta\left[\sum_{K=1}^{M}(M+1-K)^2 p_K\right] + (1-\theta)\sum_{K=1}^{M} K^2 p_K$$

$$= \theta\left[(M+1)^2 - 2(M+1)\mu\right] + \sum_{K=1}^{M} K^2 p_K,$$

then

$$V_R(z_k) = E_R(z_k^2) - E_R^2(z_k)$$

$$= \theta\left[(M+1)^2 - 2(M+1)\mu\right] + \sum_{K=1}^{M} K^2 p_K$$

$$-\theta^2\left[(M+1)^2 + 4\mu^2 - 4(M+1)\mu\right] - \mu^2 - 2\theta(M+1-2\mu)\mu$$

$$= \theta(1-\theta)(M+1-2\mu)^2 + \sum_{K=1}^{M} K^2 p_K - \mu^2$$

$$= \theta(1-\theta)(M+1-2\mu)^2 + \sigma^2, \ \forall \ k = 1, \ldots, n,$$

where $\sigma^2 = \sum K^2 p_K - \mu^2$. So,

$$V_R(r_k) = \theta(1-\theta) + \frac{\sigma^2}{n(M+1-2\mu)^2}.$$

Thus, on taking

$$\bar{r} = \frac{1}{n}\sum_{k=1}^{n} r_k$$

as an unbiased estimator for θ, we have

$$V(\bar{r}) = \frac{\theta(1-\theta)}{n} + \frac{\sigma^2}{n(M+1-2\mu)^2}.$$

An unbiased estimator for this $V(\bar{r})$ is

$$v(\bar{r}) = \frac{\bar{r}(1-\bar{r})}{n-1} + \frac{\sigma^2}{n(M+1-2\mu)^2}.$$

In case $M = 2$, then writing $p_1 = p$, $p_2 = 1 - p$, one gets $\mu = 2 - p$, $\sigma^2 = p(1-p)$,

4.3 Related Estimation in SRSWR and Sophisticated Sampling

$$V(\bar{r}) = \frac{\theta(1-\theta)}{n} + \frac{p(1-p)}{n(2p-1)^2}$$

and

$$v(\bar{r}) = \frac{\bar{r}(1-\bar{r})}{n-1} + \frac{p(1-p)}{n(2p-1)^2}.$$

Thus, Christofides' (2003) randomized response device reduces to Warner's (1965) randomized response device itself. If a general sampling design with positive π_i, π_{ij}-values is adopted, then for the Christofides' (2003) randomized response device the data from a sample s may be gathered as

$$z_i = \begin{cases} M - K + 1 & \text{if } i \text{ bears } A \\ K & \text{if } i \text{ bears } A^c. \end{cases}$$

Then,

$$E_R(z_i) = y_i(M + 1 - \mu) + (1 - y_i)\mu, \ i \in s$$
$$= (M + 1 - 2\mu)y_i + \mu.$$

Let

$$r_i = \frac{z_i - \mu}{M + 1 - 2\mu}.$$

Then, $E_R(r_i) = y_i$, $i \in s$. Also,

$$E_R(z_i^2) = y_i \left[(M+1)^2 + \sum K^2 p_K - 2(M+1)\sum K p_K\right] + (1-y_i)\sum K^2 p_K.$$

Noting that $y_i^2 = y_i$,

$$V_R(z_i) = E_R(z_i^2) - E_R^2(z_i)$$
$$= y_i \left[(M+1)^2 - 2(M+1)\mu\right] + \sum K^2 p_K$$
$$\quad - y_i[(M+1) - 2\mu]^2 - \mu^2 - 2y_i[(M+1) - 2\mu]\mu$$
$$= \sum K^2 p_K - \mu^2$$
$$= \sigma^2, \ \forall \ i \in U.$$

So,

$$V_R(r_i) = \frac{\sigma^2}{(M+1-2\mu)^2} = V_i,$$

say. Now,
$$e = \frac{1}{N} \sum_{i \in s} \frac{r_i}{\pi_i}$$

may be taken as an unbiased estimator for θ. Its variance is

$$V(e) = \frac{1}{N^2} \left[\sum_i \sum_{j,j>i} (\pi_i \pi_j - \pi_{ij}) \left(\frac{y_i}{\pi_i} - \frac{y_j}{\pi_j} \right)^2 + \sum_{i=1}^{N} \frac{V_i}{\pi_i} \right]$$

and

$$v(e) = \frac{1}{N^2} \left[\sum_{i \in s} \sum_{j \in s, j>i} \left(\frac{\pi_i \pi_j - \pi_{ij}}{\pi_{ij}} \right) \left(\frac{r_i}{\pi_i} - \frac{r_j}{\pi_j} \right)^2 + \sum \frac{V_i}{\pi_i} \right]$$

is an unbiased estimator for $V(e)$. Since V_i is known, it need not be estimated. If a sample s is chosen by the Rao–Hartley–Cochran (1962) scheme and the randomized responses be gathered according to the Christofides' (2003) randomized response device then, as before r_i, V_i are gathered. Naturally

$$e_{RHC} = \frac{1}{N} \sum_n r_i \frac{Q_i}{P_i}$$

provides an unbiased estimator for θ and

$$V(e_{RHC}) = \frac{1}{N^2} \left[C \sum_i \sum_{j,j>i} P_i P_j \left(\frac{y_i}{\pi_i} - \frac{y_j}{\pi_j} \right)^2 + \sum_n V_i \frac{Q_i}{P_i} \right]$$

of which an unbiased estimator is

$$v(e_{RHC}) = \frac{1}{N^2} \left[D \sum_n \sum_{n'} Q_i Q_{i'} \left(\frac{r_i}{\pi_i} - \frac{r_{i'}}{\pi_{i'}} \right)^2 + \sum_n V_i \frac{Q_i}{P_i} \right].$$

Remark 4.1. If a sample is already chosen following a specific design, the error may be controlled in different manners by drawing the randomized response data by various devices. This is because the randomized response-based variance of the transformed randomized response observations V_i-terms directly occur in the variance formula for the estimator chosen for θ. The estimated coefficient of variation also affects the measure of accuracy differently as the V_i or v_i term occurs in the estimator for the variance of the estimator of θ.

4.4 Certain Alternative RR Procedures with Rationales

Randomized response devices subsequent to Warner's (1965) pioneering one were invented principally to offer more accurate estimation procedures and partially as alternative policy measures allowing A^c, as aligned to A, also to be stigmatizing. Also, avoiding dichotomy, polychotomous attributes are also cared for. We believe enough has been covered relating to the latter by Chaudhuri and Mukerjee (1988). We need not spare additional space for them here because subsequent research does not seem to be rich enough on them.

Most of the novelty in research on single attributes that started with Chaudhuri's (2001a, 2001b) extension to unequal probability sampling was necessitated to cater to the needs of agencies busy to survey in traditional ways employing Probability Proportional to Size and Simple Random Sampling Without Replacement if they intend to cover sensitive issues as well, along with the innocuous ones in the same survey project.

Let us narrate them briefly chronologically as far as practicable.

4.4.1 Dalenius and Vitale (1974) Approach

Dalenius and Vitale (1974) considered estimating the mean of a quantitative variable which is not intrinsically stigmatizing but people are usually uncomfortable to give out truthful responses when faced with relevant queries concerned. For example, an investigator may like to properly estimate the areas of total farmlands possessed by the people in a given district of interest. Presuming the people may be reluctant to truthfully respond on such queries, Dalenius and Vitale (1974) elegantly formulated this as a problem for addressing a Qualitative Data related randomized response problem in the following manner. Supposing the true response values could be summarized into a frequency distribution with well-defined continuous class-intervals with a common width for each, they formulated the following. Each sampled respondent is offered a small instrument like a watch with a rotatable metallic hand at its center and along the perimeter of the circular disk sections are marked successively $0, 1, 2, \ldots, M$ at equal distances apart. On rotation, the metal hand is supposed after a few whirls to stop at some space between sections $(j - 1)$ and j $(j = 1, \ldots, M)$.

The person is just to say "Yes" if the class out of these M classes signified by the respective sections in the disk to which the respondent belongs is greater than the section where the rotating "hand" stops. The response should be "No" in the contrary case. For such a randomized response from any person i, say sampled, may be taken as

$$I_i = \begin{cases} 1 \text{ if } i \text{ says "Yes"} \\ 0 \text{ if } i \text{ says "No"}. \end{cases}$$

Let in $U = (1, \ldots, i, \ldots, N)$ the population of persons to be studied and f_j be the unknown number of persons in the j-th class ($j = 1, \ldots, M$) noted above. Also, let

$$\theta_j = \frac{f_j}{\sum_{j=1}^{M} f_j}$$

be the relative frequency of the j-th class. Then Dalenius and Vitale (1974) considered estimating the mean

$$\mu = \frac{\sum_{j=1}^{M} j f_j}{\sum_{j=1}^{M} f_j} = \sum_{j=1}^{M} j \theta_j.$$

Now,

$$E_R(I_i) = \frac{1}{M} \left[\sum_{j=1}^{M} j \theta_j \right] = \frac{\mu}{M}, \ \forall \, i \in U,$$

so MI_i unbiasedly estimates μ for every i in the sample.

Let us denote by λ the probability of obtaining a "Yes" response. Then,

$$\lambda = E_R(I_i) = \frac{\mu}{M}, \ \forall \, i \in U.$$

So, if λ can be unbiasedly estimated from a sample of "Yes–No" responses as $\hat{\lambda}$, say, then μ may be unbiasedly estimated by $M\hat{\lambda}$. Again,

$$\begin{aligned} V_R(I_i) &= E_R(I_i)(1 - E_R(I_i)) \\ &= \frac{\mu}{M}\left(1 - \frac{\mu}{M}\right) \\ &= \lambda(1-\lambda), \ \forall \, i \in U \\ &= V, \end{aligned}$$

say. If a simple random sample with replacement in n draws is taken, then, writing the "Yes"-response, I_k from one chosen on the k-th draw

$$\bar{I} = \frac{1}{n} \sum_{k=1}^{n} I_k = \hat{\lambda},$$

say, is an unbiased estimator for $\lambda = \mu/M$. Its variance is

$$V(\bar{I}) = \frac{\lambda(1-\lambda)}{n}.$$

4.4 Certain Alternative RR Procedures with Rationales

So,

$$v(\bar{I}) = \frac{\hat{\lambda}(1-\hat{\lambda})}{n-1}$$

unbiasedly estimates $V(\bar{I})$. To proceed for a general sampling scheme with positive inclusion probabilities π_i, π_{ij}, the Horvitz–Thompson (1952) type unbiased estimator for $\lambda = \mu/M$ is

$$e_{HT} = \frac{1}{N} \sum_{i \in s} \frac{I_i}{\pi_i}.$$

Also,

$$V(e_{HT}) = V_R E_p(e_{HT}) + E_R V_p(e_{HT}).$$

It follows easily that

$$V(e_{HT}) = \frac{1}{N^2} \left[\lambda^2 \sum_i \sum_{j,j>i} (\pi_i \pi_j - \pi_{ij}) \left(\frac{1}{\pi_i} - \frac{1}{\pi_j}\right)^2 + V \sum_{i=1}^N \frac{1}{\pi_i} \right].$$

Since λ^2 and V are unknown, unbiased estimation of $V(e_{HT})$ is not easy. We need to adopt Chaudhuri's (2002) approach in this context. From each sampled person i let us obtain two independently elicited randomized responses as I_i, J_i with an identical distribution, J_i being gathered exactly in the same manner as I_i itself. Let

$$T_i = \frac{1}{2}(I_i + J_i).$$

Then,

$$E_R(I_i) = \lambda = E_R(J_i) = \frac{\mu}{M}, \quad \forall i \in U,$$

$$V_R(I_i) = \lambda(1-\lambda) = V_R(J_i), \quad \forall i \in U,$$

$$E_R(T_i) = \lambda, \quad V_R(T_i) = \frac{V}{2}, \quad \forall i \in U.$$

So, instead of e_{HT} above, now we recommend taking for $\lambda = \mu/M$ the unbiased estimator

$$\bar{e}_{HT} = \frac{1}{N} \sum_{i \in s} \frac{T_i}{\pi_i}.$$

Its variance is then

$$V(\bar{e}_{HT}) = \frac{1}{N^2} \left[\frac{\lambda^2}{4} \sum_i \sum_{j,j>i} (\pi_i \pi_j - \pi_{ij}) \left(\frac{1}{\pi_i} - \frac{1}{\pi_j} \right)^2 + \frac{V}{2} \sum_{i=1}^N \frac{1}{\pi_i} \right].$$

Now,

$$E_R(I_i - J_i)^2 = E_R[(I_i - \lambda) - (J_i - \lambda)]^2 = 2V.$$

So,

$$\frac{1}{N} \sum_{i \in s} \frac{(I_i - J_i)^2}{4\pi_i}$$

is an unbiased estimator for $V/2$. Also, $E_R(I_i J_i) = \lambda^2$. So,

$$\frac{1}{N} \sum_{i \in s} \frac{I_i J_i}{4\pi_i}$$

is an unbiased estimator for $\lambda^2/4$. Thus,

$$v(\bar{e}_{HT}) = \frac{1}{N^2} \left[\sum_{i \in s} \frac{I_i J_i}{4\pi_i} \sum_i \sum_{j,j>i} (\pi_i \pi_j - \pi_{ij}) \left(\frac{1}{\pi_i} - \frac{1}{\pi_j} \right)^2 \right.$$
$$\left. + \frac{1}{N} \sum_{i \in s} \frac{(I_i - J_i)^2}{4\pi_i} \sum_{i \in s} \frac{1}{\pi_i} \right],$$

which is equal to

$$\frac{1}{4} \left[\frac{N-n}{n^2 N} \left(\sum_{i \in s} I_i J_i \right) \sum_i \sum_{j,j>i} (I_i - J_i)^2 + \frac{1}{nN} \sum_{i \in s} (I_i - J_i)^2 \right]$$

in case of SRSWOR, unbiasedly estimates $V(\bar{e}_{HT})$.

Finally, let us restore this solution on a "Qualitative-trait"-related randomized response to the original "Quantitative" one. Dalenius and Vitale (1974) started with a quantitative variable with its values arranged in a frequency distribution with the unknowable class-frequencies for the j-th ($j = 1, \ldots, M$) classes with x_j as the respective class-marks i.e., mid-values of the class intervals. Choosing a suitable point C and a common width h for the class-intervals, let

4.4 Certain Alternative RR Procedures with Rationales

$$\delta_j = \left(\frac{x_j - C}{h}\right), \quad j = 1, \ldots, M.$$

Then the mean μ_x of x to be estimated is

$$\mu_x = C + h \frac{\sum_{j=1}^{M} \delta_j f_j}{\sum_{j=1}^{M} f_j} = C + h\mu.$$

Since $\lambda = \mu/M$ is already estimated by $\hat{\lambda}$, our unbiased estimator for μ_x is

$$\hat{\mu}_x = C + Mh\hat{\lambda}.$$

Clearly, an unbiased estimator for the variance of $\hat{\mu}_x$ follows immediately, as

$$(Mh)^2 v\left(\bar{I}\right) = \frac{(Mh)^2 \hat{\lambda}\left(1 - \hat{\lambda}\right)}{n-1}$$

in case of SRSWR, $(Mh)^2 v\left(\bar{e}_{HT}\right)$ for general sampling scheme, and $(Mh)^2$ times the version of $v\left(\bar{e}_{HT}\right)$ for SRSWOR.

4.4.2 Liu, Chow, and Mosley's (1975) RR Device

Here the problem addressed is to estimate the proportions θ_j ($j = 1, \ldots, M$) of people in a community bearing several distinguishable traits labeled ($j = 1, \ldots, M$), with at least a few of them ponderable as stigmatizing. Liu et al. (1975) build a linear relation

$$\lambda_j = \sum_{K=1}^{M} p_{Kj} \theta_K$$

on defining the $\left(p_{Kj}\right)$ matrix in the following manner and then directly estimate λ_j and hence the θ_K's as well. Their randomized response device uses a flask with a long transparent neck marked $1, 2, \ldots, K, \ldots, M$ narrow enough to accommodate just one bead one on another. The m beads of M different colors numbering $m_1 \neq m_2 \neq \ldots \neq m_M$ are put into the flask closing the top edge by a stopper. The bottom edge is flat, dense, and without any hole. A person sampled is briefed to identify the color representing his/her trait, to shake the flask and turn it upside down and "report" the number on the neck pointing to the bottom-most bead of his/her color. Let

$$p_{11} = P(\text{a person of trait 1 reports 1}) = \frac{m_1}{m},$$

$$p_{23} = P(\text{a person of trait 2 reports 3}) = \left(\frac{m - m_2}{m}\right)\left(\frac{m - m_2 - 1}{m - 1}\right)\frac{m_2}{m - 2},$$

.

.

.

$$p_{jK} = P(\text{a person of trait j reports K}).$$

So, once we are able to estimate λ_j, through the above-noted randomized response device, we may gather from Chaudhuri and Mukerjee (1988) how to estimate the θ_K's exploiting the above relationships of λ_j vs θ_K through these p_{jk}'s. If a simple random sample with replacement in n draws is taken, then using the observed sample proportions $\hat{\lambda}_j$ of the "reported j"-values, λ_j is clearly estimated unbiasedly along with unbiased variance estimators thereof. This is not reproduced here from Chaudhuri and Mukerjee (1988). If a sample s is drawn by a general sampling scheme admitting positive inclusion probabilities π_i, π_{ij}, then one may check from Chaudhuri (2002) how to proceed for estimating the λ_j's. For a sampled person labeled i let

$$I_{ij} = \begin{cases} 1 & \text{if } i \text{ reports } j \text{ using Liu et al. device} \\ 0 & \text{if the report is not } j. \end{cases}$$

Let independently another identically produced report from him/her be

$$I'_{ij} = \begin{cases} 1 & \text{if } i \text{ reports } j \text{ using Liu et al. device} \\ 0 & \text{if the report is not } j. \end{cases}$$

Then,

$$\bar{I}_{ij} = \frac{1}{2}\left(I_{ij} + I'_{ij}\right)$$

has for every i

$$E_R(\bar{I}_{ij}) = \lambda_j, \quad V_j = V_R(\bar{I}_{ij}) = \frac{V_R(I_{ij})}{2},$$

$(I_{ij} - I'_{ij})^2/4$ unbiasedly estimates V_j, for all i, and $I_{ij}I'_{ij}$ unbiasedly estimates λ_j^2, for all $i \in U$. So,

$$\frac{1}{4N}\sum_{i \in s}\frac{(I_{ij} - I'_{ij})^2}{\pi_{ij}}$$

4.4 Certain Alternative RR Procedures with Rationales

will be taken as an unbiased estimator for V_j and

$$\frac{1}{N} \sum_{i \in s} \frac{I_{ij} I'_{ij}}{\pi_i}$$

will be taken to unbiasedly estimate λ_j^2, $j = 1, \ldots, M$. Finally,

$$\bar{e}_{HT}(j) = \frac{1}{N} \sum_{i \in s} \frac{\bar{I}_{ij}}{\pi_i}$$

will be used to unbiasedly estimate λ_j, for $j = 1, \ldots, M$. Then,

$$V(\bar{e}_{HT}(j)) = \frac{1}{N^2} \left[\frac{\lambda_j^2}{4} \sum_i \sum_{i',i'>i} (\pi_i \pi_{i'} - \pi_{ii'}) \left(\frac{\bar{I}_{ij}}{\pi_i} - \frac{\bar{I}_{i'i}}{\pi_{i'}} \right)^2 + \frac{V_j}{2} \sum_{i=1}^{N} \frac{\bar{I}_{ij}}{\pi_i} \right],$$

equal to

$$\frac{1}{N} \left[\frac{\lambda_j^2}{4} \frac{N-n}{nN(N-1)} \sum_i \sum_{i',i'>i} (I_{ij} - I_{i'j})^2 + \frac{V_j}{2n} \sum_{i=1}^{N} I_{ij} \right]$$

for SRSWOR and

$$v(\bar{e}_{HT}(j)) = \frac{1}{N^2} \left[\frac{1}{4} \sum_{i \in s} \frac{(I_{ij} I'_{ij})}{\pi_i} \sum_{i \in s} \sum_{i' \in s, i'>i} \left(\frac{\pi_i \pi_{i'} - \pi_{ii'}}{\pi_{ii'}} \right) \left(\frac{\bar{I}_{ij}}{\pi_i} - \frac{\bar{I}'_{i'i}}{\pi_{i'}} \right)^2 \right.$$

$$\left. + \frac{1}{8} \sum_{i \in s} \frac{(I_{ij} - I'_{i'j})^2}{\pi_i} \sum_{i \in s} \frac{I'_{i'j}}{\pi_i} \right],$$

equal to

$$\frac{N-n}{4n^3(n-1)} \left(\sum_{i \in s} I_{ij} I'_{ij} \right) \sum_{i \in s} \sum_{i' \in s, i'>i} (I_{ij} - I'_{i'j})^2 + \frac{1}{8n^2} \sum_{i \in s} \sum_{i' \in s, i'>i} (I_{ij} - I'_{ij})^2 \left(\sum_{i \in s} I'_{ij} \right)$$

for SRSWOR, is an unbiased estimator for $V(\bar{e}_{HT}(j))$, $j = 1, \ldots, M$.

4.4.3 Mangat and Singh's (1990) RR Device

In order to appropriately estimate the unknown proportion θ of people with a sensitive attribute in a community, Mangat and Singh (1990) slightly alter as follows the randomized response device of Warner (1965). A sampled person is offered two boxes of cards. In the first box a known proportion T $(0 < T < 1)$ of cards is marked "True" and the remaining ones marked "RR." One card is to be drawn, noticed, and returned to the box. If the card drawn is marked "True," then the respondent should respond "Yes" if he/she belongs to the sensitive category and "No" if not. If the card drawn is marked "RR," then the respondent must use the second box and draw a card out of it. This second box contains a proportion p $(0 < p < 1, p \neq 0.5)$ of cards marked A and the remaining ones marked A^c. If the card drawn out of the second box matches his/her status as related to the stigmatizing characteristic, he/she must respond "Yes," otherwise a "No" response must be provided. Of course, the entire procedure takes place outside the view of the interviewer.

The randomized response from a person labeled i is supposed to be the following:

$$z_i = \begin{cases} y_i & \text{if a "True" marked card from the first box is drawn} \\ I_i & \text{if an "RR" marked card is drawn.} \end{cases}$$

where

$$I_i = \begin{cases} 1 & \text{if the "card type" } A \text{ or } A^c \text{ "matches" the genuine trait } A \text{ or } A^c \\ 0 & \text{if a "mismatch" is observed.} \end{cases}$$

Then,

$$E_R(z_i) = Ty_i(1-T)[py_i + (1-p)(1-y_i)]$$
$$= (1-T)(1-p) + y_i[T + (1-T)(2p-1)].$$

Clearly,

$$r_i = \frac{z_i - (1-T)(1-p)}{T + (1-T)(2p-1)}$$

satisfies $E_R(r_i) = y_i$, assuming $T + (1-T)(2p-1) \neq 0$. Since the variables y_i, I_i, z_i take on only the values 0 and 1, one gets

$$V_R(z_i) = E_R(z_i)(1 - E_R(z_i))$$

and hence

$$V_R(r_i) = (1-T)(1-p)[T + p(1-T)], \forall i.$$

The subsequent study mimics that of Warner's.

4.4.4 Mangat's (1992) RR Device as Modified by Chaudhuri (2011)

Mangat's (1992) approach is a follow-up of Mangat and Singh's (1990) amendment applied on Warner's (1965) device. Mangat (1992) used the first box with cards marked "True" and "RR" in proportions $T : (1 - T)$, $(0 < T < 1)$. A person drawing a "True" marked card is to give out the truth about bearing A or A^c. One drawing an "RR" marked card is to apply now Simmons's device by drawing a card from a second box with cards marked A and B in proportions $p : (1 - p)$, $(0 < p < 1)$. If an A marked card is now drawn the truthful response will be about bearing the sensitive attribute A and otherwise about B. The true proportion θ $(0 < \theta < 1)$ of people bearing A is to be estimated but the proportion ψ of people bearing the innocuous trait B unrelated to A is supposed to be known. Treating the more realistic case of ψ being unknown, Chaudhuri (2011) amends this randomized response device of Mangat (1992) by demanding a person drawing an "RR" marked card from the first box to use independently two separate boxes—the second one containing A and B- marked cards in proportions $p_1 : (1 - p_1)$, $(0 < p_1 < 1)$ and the third box containing A and B-marked cards in proportions $p_2 : (1 - p_2)$, $(0 < p_2 < 1)$, $p_1 \neq p_2$. Responses will independently emerge about bearing A or B using similarly the second and the third box if guided to do so depending on the outcome of the draw from the first box. We then need the following:

$$y_i = \begin{cases} 1 & \text{if } i \text{ bears } A \\ 0 & \text{if } i \text{ bears } A^c. \end{cases}$$

and

$$x_i = \begin{cases} 1 & \text{if } i \text{ bears } B \\ 0 & \text{if } i \text{ bears } B^c. \end{cases}$$

Finally,

$$I_i = \begin{cases} 1 & \text{if the type of card drawn from the second box matches trait } A \text{ or } B \\ 0 & \text{if the type of card drawn from the second box does not match trait } A \text{ or } B. \end{cases}$$

and

$$J_i = \begin{cases} 1 & \text{if the type of card drawn from the third box matches trait } A \text{ or } B \\ 0 & \text{if the type of card drawn from the third box does not match trait } A \text{ or } B. \end{cases}$$

Then,

$$E_R(I_i) = Ty_i + (1-T)[p_1 y_i + (1-p_1) x_i],$$

$$E_R(J_i) = Ty_i + (1-T)[p_2 y_i + (1-p_2) x_i],$$

and,

$$E_R[(1-p_2) I_i - (1-p_1) J_i] = (p_1 - p_2) y_i.$$

So,

$$r_i = \frac{(1-p_2) I_i - (1-p_1) J_i}{p_1 - p_2}$$

has

$$E_R(r_i) = y_i, \quad V_R(r_i) = E_R[r_i(r_i - 1)],$$

since $y_i^2 = y_i$. Therefore, $r_i(r_i - 1)$ unbiasedly estimates $V_R(r_i) = V_i$. Thus, on taking a sample by

- simple random sampling with replacement,
- general scheme with positive inclusion probabilities π_i, π_{ij},
- the Rao et al. (1962) scheme or
- SRSWOR,

estimation of θ along with estimated standard error and a coefficient of variation is a simple matter indeed.

4.4.5 Mangat, Singh, and Singh's (1992) Device

The Mangat, Singh, and Singh (1992) technique came yet again as a modification of Mangat's (1992) extension of Simmon's Unrelated Question Model. As Mangat (1992) himself, these three colleagues noted above restricted to simple random sampling with replacement alone. But in keeping with our stand to emphasize that a randomized response device works independently of how a sample is taken, let us demonstrate the essence of this device with its genesis in Mangat et al. (1992) works. For details see Chaudhuri (2011).

Let

$$y_i = \begin{cases} 1 & \text{if } i \text{ bears } A \\ 0 & \text{if } i \text{ bears } A^c, \end{cases}$$

and

$$x_i = \begin{cases} 1 & \text{if } i \text{ bears } B \\ 0 & \text{if } i \text{ bears } B^c. \end{cases}$$

4.4 Certain Alternative RR Procedures with Rationales

A is stigmatizing and our mission is to estimate θ, the proportion bearing A in a community, B is an innocuous attribute unrelated to A with an unknown proportion ψ of people bearing it. Three boxes containing cards are presented to a sample person labeled i.

He/she is requested to draw a card from the first box. Without showing it to the investigator he/she is to give out the true value y_i if A is his/her true trait; if not, he/she is to draw a card from the second box; this box contains cards marked A, B in proportions $p_1 : (1 - p_1)$, $(0 < p_1 < 1)$; he/she is to report the value x_i if a B-type card is chosen and he/she bears B; else he/she is to report "No." He/she is to repeat the exercise with the third box with A and B-marked cards in proportions $p_2 : (1 - p_2)$, $(0 < p_2 < 1, p_2 \neq p_1)$, if so guided by the outcome of the exercise with the first box. Let

$$I_i = \begin{cases} 1 \text{ if a "Yes" results through the second box trial} \\ 0 \text{ if a "No" results through the second box trial.} \end{cases}$$

and

$$J_i = \begin{cases} 1 \text{ if a "Yes" results through the third box trial} \\ 0 \text{ if a "No" results through the third box trial.} \end{cases}$$

Then,

$$E_R(I_i) = y_i + (1 - y_i)(1 - p_1)x_i,$$

$$E_R(J_i) = y_i + (1 - y_i)(1 - p_2)x_i.$$

Hence,

$$r_i = \frac{(1 - p_2)I_i - (1 - p_1)J_i}{p_1 - p_2}$$

gives $E_R(r_i) = y_i$ and $V_R(r_i) = V_i = E_R(r_i(r_i - 1))$ giving $v_i = r_i(r_i - 1)$ as an unbiased estimator for V_i. The rest follows as usual.

4.4.6 Mangat's (1994) Device

Mangat (1994) gave the following simple but efficient randomized response device. A person bearing A is to truthfully say so. If he/she does not belong to the stigmatizing group, he/she is to apply Warner's randomized response device. Using the device, he/she responds with a "Yes" or "No" to the statement "I belong to A" or to the statement "I belong to A^c". Mangat (1994) of course confined only to simple random sampling with replacement. But we may as follows extend it to a general sampling design with positive inclusion probabilities π_i, π_{ij} for all $i \in U$

and $i, j (i \neq j)$ in U. For this scheme of Mangat (1994), the randomized response from a person labeled i, say, is

$$I_i = \begin{cases} 1 \text{ if a "Yes" results through the procedure} \\ 0 \text{ if a "No" results through the procedure.} \end{cases}$$

Then

$$E_R(I_i) = y_i + (1 - y_i)(1 - p) = (1 - p) + py_i.$$

Obviously,

$$r_i = \frac{I_i - (1 - p)}{p}$$

has $E_R(r_i) = y_i$. Then, since $y_i^2 = y_i$

$$\begin{aligned} V_R(r_i) &= \frac{V_R(I_i)}{p^2} \\ &= \frac{E_R(I_i)(1 - E_R(I_i))}{p^2} \\ &= \left(\frac{1-p}{p}\right)(1 - y_i) \\ &= V_i \end{aligned}$$

say. Then,

$$v_i = \left(\frac{1-p}{p}\right)(1 - r_i)$$

is an unbiased estimator for $V_i, i \in U$.

A subsequent development follows as a routine. We choose to omit the details to save space. Mangat (1994) himself only covered the theory based on simple random sampling with replacement alone. We need not reproduce his work here. We discussed earlier how to compare relative efficacies of contesting randomized response procedures based on competing sampling designs combined with linear estimators involving direct responses and their derived versions with randomized responses, instead of direct responses for sensitive issues. Comparisons are generally hard to be convincing.

4.4.7 Singh and Joarder's (1997a) RR Device

The basics of the Singh and Joarder's (1997a) device are the same as in Warner's (1965) randomized response device. But the difference is as follows.

4.4 Certain Alternative RR Procedures with Rationales

If a person labeled i bears A^c is to say so if so guided by a card drawn from a box of A and A^c marked cards in proportions $p : (1-p)$, $(0 < p < 1)$. However, if he/she bears A and is directed by the card to admit that, he/she is advised to postpone the reporting based on the first draw of the card from the box but to report on the basis of a second draw. So, writing

$$I_i = \begin{cases} 1 \text{ if person } i \text{ responds "Yes" following Singh and Joarder's instructions} \\ 0 \text{ if person } i \text{ responds "No" following Singh and Joarder's instructions.} \end{cases}$$

Then,

$$E_R(I_i) = (1-p)(1-y_i) + y_i[(1-p)p + p]$$
$$= (1-p) + y_i[(2p-1) + p(1-p)],$$

and

$$r_i = \frac{I_i - (1-p)}{(2p-1) + p(1-p)}$$

satisfies $E_R(r_i) = y_i$. Since $y_i = y_i^2$ it follows that

$$V_i = V_R(r_i) = E_R[r_i(r_i - 1)]$$

and hence $v_i = r_i(r_i - 1)$ is an unbiased estimator for V_i, $i \in U$. An alternative formula for V_i and hence of v_i is given by Chaudhuri (2011, p 56).

4.4.8 Randomized Response Using the Poisson Distribution

Frequently, the sensitive attribute is very rare and only a small number of people belong to the stigmatizing category. For example, the number of terminated pregnancies due to rape, or the number of children who are victims of sex violence in the family. In cases such as the ones previously mentioned, a huge sample size would be required to estimate the number (and population proportion) of people having the sensitive characteristic. Modern technology enables the collection of information from a large sample of people, via the Internet, email, or the telephone. In case of a very rare sensitive attribute, Land, Singh, and Sedory (2012) propose the use of the Poisson distribution. We briefly describe their approach in what follows.

Let θ_1 be the proportion of people having the sensitive attribute A_1. Assume that a large simple random sample of size n is selected from the population with replacement, such that as $n \to \infty$, $\theta_1 \to 0$, but $n\theta_1 = \lambda_1$, with λ_1 finite. Consider now a rare nonstigmatizing attribute A_2 which is unrelated to A_1. Let θ_2 be the population proportion of people having the characteristic A_2 and assume $n \to \infty$,

$\theta_2 \to 0$, but $n\theta_2 = \lambda_2$, with λ_2 finite and known. Each sampled person is requested to truthfully respond with a "Yes" or "No" to one of the following two questions:

(I) Do you possess the rare sensitive attribute A_1?
(II) Do you possess the rare nonsensitive attribute A_2?

Respondents provide an answer to (I) with probability p and to (II) with probability $1 - p$ with the use of a randomization device. Of course, in the case of collecting the information via telephone or the Internet (which is the most plausible scenario given the large sample size) the use of a randomization device is out of question. Instead a randomization takes place without a device. For example, a participant could be requested to respond to (I) if say, he/she was born in the months of April through July and to (II) otherwise. The probability of a "Yes" response is obviously

$$\theta_0 = p\theta_1 + (1-p)\theta_2.$$

Given that both attributes A_1 and A_2 are very rare, then one can assume that as $n \to \infty$ and $\theta_0 \to 0$, then $n\theta_0 = \lambda_0$ with

$$\lambda_0 = p\lambda_1 + (1-p)\lambda_2$$

being finite.

Assume now that we have a random sample $x_1, x_2, \ldots, x_n$ from the Poisson distribution with parameter λ_0. Then, the likelihood function is

$$L(\lambda_1 \mid x_1, \ldots, x_n) = \prod_{i=1}^{n} \frac{[p\lambda_1 + (1-p)\lambda_2]^{x_i}}{x_i!} \exp(-p\lambda_1 - (1-p)\lambda_2)$$

and it can be shown (by standard methods) that the maximum likelihood estimator of λ_1 is

$$\hat{\lambda}_1 = \frac{1}{p}[\bar{x} - (1-p)\lambda_2].$$

The following result can be easily established. For details, see, Land et al. (2012).

Theorem 4.1. *The estimator $\hat{\lambda}_1$ is unbiased for λ_1 with variance given by*

$$V(\hat{\lambda}_1) = \frac{\lambda_1}{np} + \frac{(1-p)\lambda_2}{np^2}.$$

An unbiased estimator for the variance is provided by the following theorem, the proof of which is straightforward.

4.4 Certain Alternative RR Procedures with Rationales

Theorem 4.2. *An unbiased estimator of the variance of λ_1 is given by*

$$\hat{V}\left(\hat{\lambda}_1\right) = \frac{\bar{x}}{np^2}.$$

The scenario described above assumes that the prevalence of the very rare unrelated characteristic A_2 is known. However, it is quite reasonable to assume that such a case is not often realistic. Thus, a modification of the above method is necessary, which we immediately describe.

Each respondent in the simple random sample of size n chosen with replacement from the population is first presented with the same two questions as above

(I) Do you possess the rare sensitive attribute A_1?
(II) Do you possess the rare non sensitive attribute A_2?

and again, each participant provides a "Yes" or "No" answer to (I) with probability p and to (II) with probability $1 - p$. Let us call this stage as the first stage of the experiment.

Next the respondent is presented with the same two questions, i.e.,

(I) Do you possess the rare sensitive attribute A_1?
(II) Do you possess the rare non sensitive attribute A_2?

but he/she provides a "Yes" or "No" answer to question (I) with probability q and to question (II) with probability $1 - q$, with $q \neq p$. Let us call this stage as the second stage of the experiment. Clearly, the probability of a "Yes" response in the first and second stage is

$$\beta_1 = p\theta_1 + (1-p)\theta_2$$

and

$$\beta_2 = q\theta_1 + (1-q)\theta_2,$$

respectively.

Assume now that as $n \to \infty$, $\beta_1 \to 0$, and $\beta_2 \to 0$, but $n\beta_1 = \lambda_1^*$ and $n\beta_2 = \lambda_2^*$ both finite. Assume that $x_1^{(1)}, x_2^{(1)}, \ldots, x_n^{(1)}$ is the random sample from the Poisson distribution with parameter λ_1^* corresponding to the first stage of the experiment and $x_1^{(2)}, x_2^{(2)}, \ldots, x_n^{(2)}$ is the random sample from the Poisson distribution with parameter λ_2^* corresponding to the second stage of the experiment. Then we have the following results, the proofs of which are given in Land et al. (2012) .

Theorem 4.3. *An unbiased estimator of the parameter λ_1 for the rare sensitive attribute A_1 is given by*

$$\hat{\lambda}_1 = \frac{1}{p-q}\left[(1-q)\bar{x}^{(1)} - (1-p)\bar{x}^{(2)}\right],$$

where $\bar{x}^{(1)}$ and $\bar{x}^{(2)}$ denote the sample mean of the first and second sample, respectively.

Theorem 4.4. *The variance of $\hat{\lambda}_1$ is given by*

$$V\left(\hat{\lambda}_1\right) = \frac{\lambda_1}{n(p-q)^2}\left[p(1-q)^2 + q(1-p)^2 - 2pq(1-p)(1-q)\right]$$

$$+ \frac{\lambda_2}{n(p-q)^2}\left[(1-p)(1-q)(2-p-q) - 2(1-p)^2(1-q)^2\right].$$

Theorem 4.5. *An unbiased estimator of the parameter λ_2 corresponding to the rare unrelated attribute A_2 is given by*

$$\hat{\lambda}_2 = \frac{1}{p-q}\left(q\bar{x}^{(1)} - p\bar{x}^{(2)}\right)$$

with variance

$$V\left(\hat{\lambda}_2\right) = \frac{\lambda_1}{n(p-q)^2}\left[pq(p+q) - 2p^2q^2\right]$$

$$+ \frac{\lambda_2}{n(p-q)^2}\left[(1-p)q^2 + (1-q)p^2 - 2pq(1-p)(1-q)\right].$$

Finally, the following result provides unbiased estimators of the variances of $\hat{\lambda}_1$ and $\hat{\lambda}_2$.

Theorem 4.6. *Unbiased estimators of the variances of $\hat{\lambda}_1$ and $\hat{\lambda}_2$ are provided by*

$$\hat{V}\left(\hat{\lambda}_1\right) = \frac{\hat{\lambda}_1}{n(p-q)^2}\left[p(1-q)^2 + q(1-p)^2 - 2pq(1-p)(1-q)\right]$$

$$+ \frac{\hat{\lambda}_2}{n(p-q)^2}\left[(1-p)(1-q)(2-p-q) - 2(1-p)^2(1-q)^2\right],$$

and

$$\hat{V}\left(\hat{\lambda}_2\right) = \frac{\hat{\lambda}_1}{n(p-q)^2}\left[pq(p+q) - 2p^2q^2\right]$$

$$+ \frac{\hat{\lambda}_2}{n(p-q)^2}\left[(1-p)q^2 + (1-q)p^2 - 2pq(1-p)(1-q)\right],$$

respectively.

The above method can be extended to cases of different sampling schemes. For example, Lee, Uhm, and Kim (2012) proposed estimators for the case of stratified sampling and stratified double sampling.

Remark 4.2. The use of the Poisson distribution has been utilized by other authors as well. For example Cruyff, Bockenholt, van der Hout, and van der Heijden (2008) consider the case of surveys with multiple sensitive questions where the number of questions applicable to a respondent is modeled according to a (truncated) Poisson distribution.

4.5 Alternative Randomized Response Generation

In a recent paper, Singh and Grewal (2013) considered a modified version of Kuk's (1990) randomized response model and demonstrated its superiority over the original model. Their approach is to utilize the geometric distribution in the following way:

Assume that we have a simple random sample of size n selected from the population with replacement. Our purpose is to estimate the population proportion θ of people having the sensitive characteristic A. Each respondent is provided with two decks of cards, just as in the usual Kuk (1990) technique. Each deck consists of only two kinds of cards. A card is either marked as an A card or an A^c card. The proportion of A cards in the first and second deck is p_1 and p_2 respectively. A respondent is instructed to use the first deck if he/she belongs to the sensitive category A, otherwise he/she is to use the second deck. The respondent is further instructed to draw cards from the deck, one-by-one with replacement until he/she gets the first card whose kind coincides with his/her status regarding the sensitive characteristic. For example, a person belonging to the stigmatizing category, draws cards from the first deck until he/she draws an A marked card. The respondent then reports just the number of times he drew a card from the deck.

Assume that X represents the number reported by a participant drawing cards from the first deck and similarly Y that represents the number reported by a person drawing from the second deck. Then X and Y follow the geometric distribution with parameter p_1 and p_2 respectively. Let Z_i represent the response provided by the i-th participant. Then Singh and Grewal (2013) showed that the quantity

$$\hat{\theta} = \frac{p_1 p_2 \bar{Z} - p_1}{p_2 - p_1}$$

is unbiased for θ, where $\bar{Z}$ represents the sample average of $Z_1, \ldots, Z_n$ and provided $p_1 \neq p_2$. The variance of the estimator is given by

$$V\left(\hat{\theta}\right) = \frac{\theta(1-\theta)}{n} + \frac{\theta p_2^2 (1-p_1) + (1-\theta) p_1^2 (1-p_2)}{n(p_2 - p_1)^2}.$$

Motivated by the work of Singh and Grewal (2013) we investigate whether the same conclusions are valid in cases of other randomized response techniques as well. In what follows we describe briefly this general approach.

As usual, assume that we need to unbiasedly estimate the proportion of people in a certain community who possess a sensitive characteristic A, like the ones described in previous chapters of this book.

Let $U = (1, \ldots, i, \ldots, N)$ denote a finite population of N labeled individuals with a stigmatizing real variable y defined on it with values $y_i, i \in U$. Let

$$y_i = \begin{cases} 1 & \text{if person } i \text{ bears } A \\ 0 & \text{if person } i \text{ bears } A^c \end{cases}$$

Also, let similarly x be another variable defined on the population U with values

$$x_i = \begin{cases} 1 & \text{if person } i \text{ bears } B \\ 0 & \text{if person } i \text{ bears } B^c \end{cases}$$

for $i \in U$. Here B stands for an innocuous characteristic unrelated to the stigmatizing characteristic A.

Assume that s is a sample drawn from U with suitable selection probability $p(s)$, on employing a sampling design p.

Let us recall that Warner's (1965) randomized response device essentially uses a box of identical cards differing only in bearing the marks A and A^c in proportions $p : (1 - p)$ where p is pre-assigned by the investigator with $0 < p < 1, p \neq 0.5$. A sampled person i draws a card from the box and announces only the number I_i where

$$I_i = \begin{cases} 1 & \text{if his/her trait matches the card type drawn} \\ 0 & \text{otherwise.} \end{cases}$$

Of course the card drawn is placed back in the box.

We adopt the Singh and Grewal (2013) approach in the following way: A sampled person i gives as a response the number g_i which is the draw number on which for the first time a match occurs for his/her trait with the card drawn in simple random sampling of one card with replacement from the box. Of course, the finally drawn card is to be returned to the box. Let us call this procedure as "Warner-Revised".

Let E_R and V_R denote the operators for the expectation and variance respectively with respect generically to the randomized response technique. Following Walpole and Myers (1993), we could write

$$E_R(g_i) = \frac{y_i}{p} + \frac{1 - y_i}{1 - p},$$

4.5 Alternative Randomized Response Generation

and

$$V_R(g_i) = \frac{y_i(1-p)}{p^2} + \frac{(1-y_i)p}{(1-p)^2}.$$

So the quantity

$$r_i = \frac{g_i - (1-p)^{-1}}{p^{-1} - (1-p)^{-1}} = \frac{p[(1-p)g_i - 1]}{1-2p}$$

has $E_R(r_i) = y_i$, i.e., r_i is an unbiased estimator for y_i with variance

$$V_R(r_i) = \frac{p^2(1-p)^2}{(1-2p)^2}\left[\frac{p}{(1-p)^2} + \frac{y_i(1-2p)(1-p+p^2)}{p^2(1-p)^2}\right]$$

$$= \frac{p^3}{(1-2p)^2} + \frac{1-p+p^2}{1-2p}y_i$$

$$= V_i,$$

say. So an unbiased estimator for V_i is

$$v_i = \frac{p^3}{(1-2p)^2} + \frac{1-p+p^2}{1-2p}r_i, \ i \in s.$$

Trivially,

$$V_i = \frac{p^3}{(1-2p)^2} \text{ if } y_i = 0$$

and

$$V_i = \frac{(1-p)^3}{(1-2p)^2} \text{ if } y_i = 1.$$

Kuk's (1990) randomized response device provides two boxes. One is to be used by a person bearing the stigmatizing characteristic A and the other by a person having the complementary characteristic A^c. The first box contains two kinds of cards, say red and blue, in proportions $p_1 : (1-p_1)$ with $0 < p_1 < 1$ and the second box the same kind of cards but in proportions $p_2 : (1-p_2)$, with $0 < p_2 < 1$ and $p_2 \neq p_1$. A sampled person i makes K $(K \geq 2)$ draws randomly with replacement one card at each draw from the appropriate box to be used. The person announces f_i which is the number of red cards drawn. Again, the last drawn card is put back in the box.

As in the case of Warner-Revised technique, in this "Kuk-Revised" approach, the i-th sampled person's response is the draw number K_i on which a red card is drawn for the first time in successive random draws with replacement from the appropriate box, to which the finally chosen red card is returned.

For the "Kuk-Revised" randomized response technique, we may write

$$E_R(K_i) = \frac{y_i}{p_1} + \frac{1-y_i}{p_2}$$

$$= \frac{1}{p_2} + y_i\left(\frac{1}{p_1} - \frac{1}{p_2}\right)$$

$$= \frac{1}{p_2} + \left(\frac{p_2 - p_1}{p_1 p_2}\right) y_i.$$

Therefore,

$$r_i = \frac{(K_i - (1/p_2))\, p_1 p_2}{p_2 - p_1}$$

has $E_R(r_1) = y_i$, i.e., r_i unbiasedly estimates y_i. In addition,

$$V_R(K_i) = \frac{y_i(1-p_1)}{p_1^2} + \frac{(1-y_i)(1-p_2)}{p_2^2}$$

$$= \frac{1-p_2}{p_2^2} + \left[\frac{1-p_1}{p_1^2} - \frac{1-p_2}{p_2^2}\right] y_i,$$

with

$$V_R(K_i) = \frac{1-p_2}{p_2^2} \text{ if } y_1 = 0$$

and

$$V_R(K_i) = \frac{1-p_1}{p_1^2} \text{ if } y_i = 1.$$

Since

$$V_i = V_R(r_i) = \frac{p_1^2 p_2^2}{(p_2 - p_1)^2} V_R(K_i),$$

an unbiased estimator for V_i is

$$v_i = \frac{p_1^2 p_2^2}{(p_2 - p_1)^2} \left[\frac{1-p_2}{p_2^2} + \frac{(p_2 - p_1)(p_1 + p_2 - p_1 p_2)}{p_1^2 p_2^2} r_i\right], \forall\, i \in s.$$

4.5 Alternative Randomized Response Generation

In Simmons's randomized response technique as described by Horvitz et al. (1967) and Greenberg et al. (1969) and revised by Chaudhuri (2001a,b, 2011), a sampled person i chooses randomly a card from a box which contains cards marked A and B in proportions $p_1 : (1 - p_1)$, $0 < p_1 < 1$. The person's response is I_i where

$$I_i = \begin{cases} 1 & \text{if his/her trait } A \text{ or } B \text{ matches the card type drawn} \\ 0 & \text{otherwise.} \end{cases}$$

The same person draws a card from a second box which contains A and B type cards but in proportions $p_2 : (1 - p_2)$ with $0 < p_2 < 1$, $p_2 \neq p_1$ and reports the number J_i where

$$J_i = \begin{cases} 1 & \text{if his/her trait } A \text{ or } B \text{ matches the card type drawn} \\ 0 & \text{otherwise.} \end{cases}$$

For the "Simmons-Revised" randomized response model (adopting the terminology used above), person i provides two responses: The first is g_i which is the draw number when for the first time his/her trait matches the card type when cards are drawn randomly with replacement from the first box and the second is h_i which is generated following the same procedure, but for the second box. Of course, the finally drawn card from each box is to be returned to the corresponding box. Then

$$E_R(g_i) = \frac{y_i}{p_1} + \frac{x_i}{1 - p_1}, \tag{4.2}$$

$$E_R(h_i) = \frac{y_i}{p_2} + \frac{x_i}{1 - p_2}. \tag{4.3}$$

Then, from the above two equations (4.2) and (4.3) we have that

$$E_R\left(\frac{g_i}{1 - p_2} - \frac{h_i}{1 - p_1}\right) = \frac{y_i(p_2 - p_1)}{p_1 p_2 (1 - p_1)(1 - p_2)}.$$

Now let

$$r_i = \frac{p_1 p_2}{p_2 - p_1} \left[(1 - p_1) g_i - (1 - p_2) h_i\right]. \tag{4.4}$$

Then $E_R(r_i) = y_i$. In addition,

$$V_R(g_i) = \frac{y_i(1 - p_1)}{p_1^2} + \frac{x_i p_1}{(1 - p_1)^2} \tag{4.5}$$

and

$$V_R(h_i) = \frac{y_i(1-p_2)}{p_2^2} + \frac{x_i p_2}{(1-p_2)^2}. \tag{4.6}$$

Combining (4.4) with (4.5) and (4.6) one can calculate the variance of r_i by means of the following equation

$$V_i = V_R(r_i) = \frac{p_1^2 p_2^2}{(p_2-p_1)^2}\left[(1-p_1)^2 V_R(g_i) + (1-p_2)^2 V_R(h_i)\right].$$

Since y_i takes only the values zero and one, we may write

$$\begin{aligned}V_i &= E_R(r_i^2) - (E_R(r_i))^2 \\ &= E_R(r_i^2) - y_i^2 \\ &= E_R(r_i^2) - y_i \\ &= E_R(r_i^2) - E_R(r_i) \\ &= E_R[r_i(r_i-1)]\end{aligned}$$

from which it follows that $v_i = r_i(r_i - 1)$ is an unbiased estimator for V_i for all i in s.

In the remaining of this section, we present our results for estimating $Y = \sum_{i=1}^{N} y_i$ and hence for $\theta = \bar{Y} = Y/N$ as N is supposedly known, based or randomized responses for the three newly proposed randomized response devices. We assume that the sample is chosen by

1. simple random sampling without replacement (SRSWOR),
  or
2. a general sampling design p admitting positive inclusion probabilities $\pi_i = \sum_{s \ni i} p(s)$ for $i \in U$ and $\pi_{ij} = \sum_{s \ni i,j} p(s)$ for pairs $i, j \in U, i \neq j$,
  or
3. Rao et al. (1962) scheme.

By E_p, V_p we shall denote the expectation and variance operator with respect to the sampling design p and by

$$E = E_p E_R = E_R E_p$$

and

$$V = E_p V_R + V_p E_R = E_R V_p + V_R E_p$$

the overall expectation and variance operators.

4.5 Alternative Randomized Response Generation

If true values y_i were available, then the sample mean $\bar{y} = \left(\sum_{i \in s} y_i\right)/n$ based on a simple random sample of size n drawn without replacement unbiasedly estimates $\bar{Y}$ having variance

$$V_p(\bar{y}) = \frac{N-n}{nN(N-1)} \sum_{i=1}^{N} (y_i - \bar{Y})^2$$

which admits an unbiased estimator

$$v_p(\bar{y}) = \frac{N-n}{nN(n-1)} \sum_{i \in s} (y_i - \bar{y})^2.$$

When direct responses y_i are unavailable, rather only unbiased estimators r_i for y_i are available from randomized responses by any of the three randomized response techniques described above. Then, instead of $\bar{y}$, the estimator

$$\bar{r} = \frac{1}{n} \sum_{i \in s} r_i$$

will unbiasedly estimate $\theta = \bar{Y}$. Also, it will follow that

$$V(\bar{r}) = \frac{N-n}{nN(N-1)} \sum_{i=1}^{N} (y_i - \bar{Y})^2 + \frac{1}{nN} \sum_{i=1}^{N} V_i$$

which is unbiasedly estimated by

$$v(\bar{r}) = \frac{N-n}{nN(n-1)} \sum_{i \in s} (r_i - \bar{r})^2 + \frac{1}{nN} \sum_{i \in s} v_i.$$

In case of a general sampling scheme admitting positive inclusion probabilities π_i's and π_{ij}'s

$$e = \frac{1}{N} \sum_{i \in s} \frac{r_i}{\pi_i}$$

will unbiasedly estimate θ having the overall variance

$$V(e) = \frac{1}{N^2} \left[\sum_{i} \sum_{j, j > i} (\pi_i \pi_j - \pi_{ij}) \left(\frac{y_i}{\pi_i} - \frac{y_j}{\pi_j}\right)^2 + \sum_{i=1}^{N} \frac{V_i}{\pi_i} \right].$$

The variance is unbiasedly estimated by

$$v(e) = \frac{1}{N^2} \left[\sum_{i \in s} \sum_{j \in s, j > i} \left(\frac{\pi_i \pi_j - \pi_{ij}}{\pi_{ij}} \right) \left(\frac{r_i}{\pi_i} - \frac{r_j}{\pi_j} \right)^2 + \sum_{i \in s} \frac{v_i}{\pi_i} \right].$$

If a sample of n distinct units is chosen by the Rao, Hartley and Cochran Method from the population with known normed size measures P_i, with $0 < P_i < 1$ and $\sum_{i=1}^{N} P_i = 1$ and Q_i denotes summed P_i's over the i-th random group of N_i units, then

$$e_{RHC} = \frac{1}{N} \sum_n r_i \frac{Q_i}{P_i}$$

unbiasedly estimates θ. Here $\sum_n$ is the sum over the n random groups formed in implementing the Rao, Hartley and Cocharn scheme. Its variance is (see Chaudhuri, Adhikary, and Dihidar 2000)

$$V(e_{RHC}) = \frac{1}{N^2} \left[C \sum_i \sum_{j, j > i} P_i P_j \left(\frac{y_i}{P_i} - \frac{y_j}{P_j} \right)^2 + \sum_i V_i \left(\frac{1}{P_i} - 1 \right) \right]$$

where $C = \left(\sum_n N_i^2 - N \right) / (N(N-1))$. The variance is unbiasedly estimated by

$$v(e_{RHC}) = \frac{1}{N^2} \left[D \sum_n \sum_{n'} Q_i Q_{i'} \left(\frac{r_i}{P_i} - \frac{r_{i'}}{P_{i'}} \right)^2 + \sum_n v_i \frac{Q_i}{P_i} \right]$$

where $D = \left(\sum_n N_i^2 - N \right) / \left(N^2 - \sum_n N_i^2 \right)$.

In case a simple random sample with replacement is taken in n draws, we shall denote the value of y by Y_K for the person chosen on the K-th draw, $K = 1, \ldots, n$ and r_K will be such that $E_R(r_K) = Y_K$ and v_K such that $E_R(v_K) = V_K = V_R(r_K)$. Then

$$\bar{r} = \frac{1}{n} \sum_{K=1}^{n} r_K$$

will unbiasedly estimate $\bar{Y}$ and

$$V(\bar{r}) = \frac{1}{n} \left[\theta(1-\theta) + \sum_{K=1}^{n} V_K \right]$$

where

$$V_K = \frac{1}{N} \sum_{i=1}^{N} (y_i - \bar{Y})^2, \, \forall \, K = 1, \ldots, n.$$

Writing

$$s^2 = \frac{1}{n-1} \sum_{K=1}^{n} (Y_K - \bar{y})^2,$$

where $\bar{y} = \left(\sum_{K=1}^{n} Y_K\right)/n$, the variance $V(\bar{r})$ has an unbiased estimator as

$$v(\bar{r}) = \frac{1}{n-1} \left[\bar{r}(1-\bar{r}) + \sum_{K=1}^{n} (r_K - \bar{r})^2 \right].$$

Remark 4.3. Just as in the case of the approach of Singh and Grewal (2013), we can verify by numerical simulations that the revised procedures as described above are better than their classical counterparts.

Remark 4.4. Obviously the randomized responses for the original and the revised procedures are byproducts of the binomial and the geometric distribution respectively. A further development would be to use the negative binomial distribution as a randomization device. Under this scenario, respondents would be asked to report the number of cards drawn until a card matching their trait is drawn say l times. It is expected that utilizing the negative binomial distribution will give procedures which fair better that their classical counterparts. But, one may have in mind that in such a case, cooperation of the participants might be in jeopardy.

4.6 Estimation for more than one Sensitive Characteristics

In some cases we may be interested in gathering information on multiple sensitive characteristics of the same population at the same time. This information could be useful for various reasons. It may be used for weighting on post-stratification purposes. For example we might be interested in the proportion of tax evaders with income above a certain level. Or for example we might be interested in the proportion of college athletes using illegal substances and engaging in plagiarism activities. In societies where political affiliation might be considered as sensitive, we may want to weight the percentage of people who would like to vote for a certain candidate based on party affiliation. Tamhane (1981), Christofides (2005b), Moshagen and Musch (2011), Barabesi, Franceschi, and Marcheselli (2012), and Lee, Sedory, and Singh (2013) discuss the case of estimation of multiple sensitive characteristics. In this section we will briefly describe three of the most recent methods for dealing with two or more sensitive characteristics at the same time. We will avoid presenting theoretical results. The interested reader can consult the relevant references for more details.

4.6.1 Estimating Two Characteristics

Assume that we have two sensitive characteristics A and B. These two characteristics could be dependent or independent. We will assume that the two characteristics are dependent, for otherwise, one can estimate all quantities of interest by estimating the prevalence of the two characteristics separately.

Let θ_A and θ_B be the population proportion of people belonging to the stigmatizing groups A and B. Suppose that we have a random sample of size n drawn with replacement from the population. Each sampled person is provided with two randomization devices such the one described in Christofides (2003). The first randomization device produces each one of the integers $1, 2, \ldots, M_A$ with probabilities $p_1, p_2, \ldots, p_{M_A}$ such that

$$p_j > 0 \text{ for } j = 1, \ldots, M_A, \quad \sum_{j=1}^{M_A} p_j = 1 \text{ and } p_j \neq \frac{1}{M_A} \text{ for at least one } j.$$

Using the device in the absence of the interviewer, the i-th sampled person produces an integer say, k and reports the number $M_A - k + 1$ if he/she belongs to the sensitive group A, or the integer k otherwise.

The second randomization device works exactly as the first one and produces each one of the integers $1, 2, \ldots, M_B$ with probabilities $q_1, q_2, \ldots, q_{M_B}$ such that

$$q_j > 0 \text{ for } j = 1, \ldots, M_B, \quad \sum_{j=1}^{M_B} q_j = 1 \text{ and } q_j \neq \frac{1}{M_B} \text{ for at least one } j.$$

Using the device in the absence of the interviewer, the i-th sampled person produces an integer say, l and reports the number $M_B - l + 1$ if he/she belongs to the sensitive group B, or the integer l otherwise. Let z_i, w_i be the numbers reported by the i-th sampled person using the first and second device respectively. Furthermore, for $i = 1, \ldots, n$ let

$$r_i = \frac{z_i - \mu_A}{M_A + 1 - 2\mu_A}$$

and

$$t_i = \frac{w_i - \mu_B}{M_B + 1 - 2\mu_B},$$

where

$$\mu_A = \sum_{k=1}^{M_A} k p_k \text{ and } \mu_B = \sum_{k=1}^{M_B} k q_k.$$

4.6 Estimation for more than one Sensitive Characteristics

Then from Sect. 4.3 it follows that

$$\bar{r} = \frac{1}{n}\sum_{i=1}^{n} r_i \text{ and } \bar{t} = \frac{1}{n}\sum_{i=1}^{n} t_i$$

are unbiased estimators of θ_A and θ_B respectively with variances

$$V(\bar{r}) = \frac{\theta_A(1-\theta_A)}{n} + \frac{\sigma_A^2}{n(M_A+1-2\mu_A)^2}$$

and

$$V(\bar{t}) = \frac{\theta_B(1-\theta_B)}{n} + \frac{\sigma_B^2}{n(M_B+1-2\mu_B)^2}$$

where

$$\sigma_A^2 = \sum_{k=1}^{M_A} k^2 p_k - \mu_A^2 \text{ and } \sigma_B^2 = \sum_{k=1}^{M_B} k^2 q_k - \mu_B^2.$$

The above two estimators alone do not give any information on quantities related to both characteristics. For example we might be interested in the following quantities:

1. The proportion θ_{AB} of people possessing both characteristics A and B.
2. The proportion $\theta_{A|B}$ of people possessing the characteristic A among those possessing the characteristic B.
3. The proportion $\theta_{A|B^c}$ of people possessing the characteristic A among those who do not possess the characteristic B.
4. The quantities in (2) and (3) but with A and B interchanged.

Observe that all other relevant quantities, can be estimated as soon as we have estimators for the above parameters. For example, the proportion of people not belonging to the sensitive group A among those belonging to the sensitive group B can be estimated by $1 - \hat{\theta}_{A|B}$ where $\hat{\theta}_{A|B}$ is an estimator of $\theta_{A|B}$. Let

$$C_A = M_A + 1 - 2\mu_A, \quad C_B = M_B + 1 - 2\mu_B,$$

$$\bar{z} = \frac{1}{n}\sum_{i=1}^{n} z_i, \quad \bar{w} = \frac{1}{n}\sum_{i=1}^{n} w_i, \quad \bar{x} = \frac{1}{n}\sum_{i=1}^{n} x_i$$

where $x_i = z_i w_i$, $i = 1, \ldots, n$.

The following results can be found in Christofides (2005b).

Theorem 4.7. *Let $\hat{\theta}_{AB} = C_A^{-1} C_B^{-1} (\bar{x} - \bar{z}\mu_B - \bar{w}\mu_A + \mu_A \mu_B)$. Then $\hat{\theta}_{AB}$ is unbiased for θ_{AB} with variance*

$$V\left(\hat{\theta}_{AB}\right) = \frac{1}{n} \left[\theta_{AB} (1 - \theta_{AB}) + \theta_A \sigma_B^2 C_B^{-2} + \theta_B \sigma_A^2 C_A^{-2} + \sigma_A^2 \sigma_B^2 C_A^{-2} C_B^{-2} \right].$$

An unbiased estimator of the variance is given by

$$\hat{V}\left(\hat{\theta}_{AB}\right) = \frac{1}{n-1} \left[\hat{\theta}_{AB} \left(1 - \hat{\theta}_{AB}\right) + \hat{\theta}_A \sigma_B^2 C_B^{-2} + \hat{\theta}_B \sigma_A^2 C_A^{-2} + \sigma_A^2 \sigma_B^2 C_A^{-2} C_B^{-2} \right].$$

Observe that an alternative form of the estimator $\hat{\theta}_{AB}$ is the following

$$\hat{\theta}_{AB} = C_A^{-1} C_B^{-1} \frac{1}{n} \sum_{i=1}^{n} (z_i - \mu_A)(w_i - \mu_B). \tag{4.7}$$

From the previous theorem it follows that a natural estimator for $\theta_{A|B}$ is the estimator

$$\hat{\theta}_{A|B} = \frac{\hat{\theta}_{AB}}{\hat{\theta}_B} = \frac{C_A^{-1} (\bar{x} - \bar{z}\mu_B - \bar{w}\mu_A + \mu_A \mu_B)}{\bar{w} - \mu_B}.$$

In view of (4.7) the estimator can also be written as

$$\hat{\theta}_{A|B} = \frac{C_A^{-1} \sum_{i=1}^{n} (z_i - \mu_A)(w_i - \mu_B)}{\sum_{i=1}^{n} (w_i - \mu_B)}.$$

Observe that $\hat{\theta}_{AB}$ is a ratio estimator and as such, it is not unbiased in general. However, the dominating term of its bias is given by the following result.

Theorem 4.8. *The bias of the estimator $\hat{\theta}_{A|B}$ is approximately*

$$E\left(\hat{\theta}_{A|B} - \theta_{A|B}\right) \approx \frac{1}{n} \sigma_B^2 C_B^{-2} \theta_B^{-3} (\theta_{AB} - \theta_A \theta_B).$$

As for the variance of the estimator, for large sample size n, we can have an approximate expression.

Theorem 4.9. *For large sample size n, the variance of the estimator $\hat{\theta}_{A|B}$ is approximately*

$$V\left(\hat{\theta}_{A|B}\right) \approx \frac{1}{n\theta_B^2} \left[\theta_{AB}(1 - \theta_{A|B}) + \left(\theta_A + \theta_{A|B}^2 - 2\theta_{A|B}\theta_A\right) \sigma_B^2 C_B^{-2} \right.$$
$$\left. + \theta_B \sigma_A^2 C_A^{-2} + \sigma_A^2 \sigma_B^2 C_A^{-2} C_B^{-2} \right].$$

4.6 Estimation for more than one Sensitive Characteristics

For the estimation of the parameter $\theta_{A|B^c}$, we have that a natural estimator is the quantity

$$\hat{\theta}_{A|B^c} = \frac{\hat{\theta}_A - \hat{\theta}_{AB}}{1 - \hat{\theta}_B} = \frac{\sum_{i=1}^n C_A^{-1}(z_i - \mu_A)\left(1 - C_B^{-1}(w_i - \mu_B)\right)}{\sum_{i=1}^n \left(1 - C_B^{-1}(w_i - \mu_B)\right)}.$$

The above estimator is also a ratio estimator and therefore it is biased in general. The dominating term of its bias is given by the following result.

Theorem 4.10. *The bias of the estimator $\hat{\theta}_{A|B^c}$ is approximately*

$$E\left(\hat{\theta}_{A|B^c} - \theta_{A|B^c}\right) \approx \frac{1}{n}\sigma_B^2 C_B^{-2}\theta_{B^c}^{-3}\left(\theta_{AB^c} - \theta_A \theta_{B^c}\right).$$

As in the case of the estimation of $\theta_{A|B}$, for large sample size n, an approximate expression for the variance is

$$V\left(\hat{\theta}_{A|B^c}\right) \approx \frac{1}{n\theta_{B^c}^2}\left[\theta_{AB^c}\left(1 - \theta_{A|B^c}\right) + \left(\theta_A + \theta_{A|B^c}^2 - 2\theta_{A|B^c}\theta_A\right)\sigma_B^2 C_B^{-2} \right.$$
$$\left. + \theta_{B^c}\sigma_A^2 C_A^{-2} + \sigma_A^2\sigma_B^2 C_A^{-2} C_B^{-2}\right].$$

In the previously described method, we assume that each sampled person is provided with two different randomization devices. However, the two devices could be identical, i.e., each participant is provided with just one randomization device to be used twice.

4.6.2 The Crossed Model

A somewhat different approach for the case of two stigmatizing characteristics is presented by Lee et al. (2013). Two models are presented, namely the Simple Model and the Crossed Model. We will say nothing about the Simple Model, given that it is a special case of the model of Christofides (2005b) described above.

For the Crossed Model, assume that we have a simple random sample of size n drawn with replacement from the population. Each sampled person is provided with two randomization devices which are to be used as follows:

Using the first randomization device the sampled person responds with "Yes" or "No" with probability P ($P \neq 0.5$) to the following question

(I) Are you a member of group A?
    and with probability $1 - P$ to the question
(II) Are you a member of group B^c?
    Using the second randomization device he/she responds with a "Yes" or "No" with probability T ($T \neq 0.5$) to the question

(III) Are you a member of group B?

and with the complementary probability $1 - T$ to the question

(IV) Are you a member of group A^c?

Clearly, a sampled person can provide any one of the following four possible responses: (Yes, Yes), (Yes, No), (No, Yes) and (No, No). Let $\lambda_{11}, \lambda_{10}, \lambda_{01}, \lambda_{00}$ be respectively the probabilities of those responses. Then it is easy to calculate that

$$\lambda_{11} = \theta_{AB}[PT + (1-P)(1-T)] - \theta_A(1-P)(1-T) - \theta_B(1-P)(1-T)$$
$$+ (1-P)(1-T)$$
$$\lambda_{10} = -\theta_{AB}[PT + (1-P)(1-T)] - \theta_A[(1-P)T - 1] - \theta_B(1-P)T + (1-P)T$$
$$\lambda_{01} = -\theta_{AB}[PT + (1-P)(1-T)] - \theta_A P(1-T) - \theta_B[P(1-T) - 1] + P(1-T)$$
$$\lambda_{00} = \theta_{AB}[PT + (1-P)(1-T)] - \theta_A PT - \theta_B PT + PT.$$

Now let $\hat{\lambda}_{11}, \hat{\lambda}_{10}, \hat{\lambda}_{01}, \hat{\lambda}_{00}$ be the sample proportions of people providing the four possible responses. Define the distance between the population proportions and the observed proportions as

$$D = \frac{1}{2} \sum_{k=0}^{1} \sum_{l=0}^{1} \left(\lambda_{kl} - \hat{\lambda}_{kl} \right)^2.$$

By minimizing this distance (by taking the partial derivatives) and by using the method of moments, unbiased estimators of $\theta_A, \theta_B, \theta_{AB}$ are obtained as follows:

$$\hat{\theta}_A = \frac{1}{2} + \frac{(T-P+1)\left(\hat{\lambda}_{11} - \hat{\lambda}_{00}\right) + (T+P-1)\left(\hat{\lambda}_{10} - \hat{\lambda}_{01}\right)}{2(P+T-1)},$$

$$\hat{\theta}_B = \frac{1}{2} + \frac{(P-T+1)\left(\hat{\lambda}_{11} - \hat{\lambda}_{00}\right) + (T+P-1)\left(\hat{\lambda}_{01} - \hat{\lambda}_{10}\right)}{2(P+T-1)},$$

$$\hat{\theta}_{AB} = \frac{PT\hat{\lambda}_{11} - (1-P)(1-T)\hat{\lambda}_{00}}{(P+T-1)[PT + (1-P)(1-T)]},$$

assuming that $P + T \neq 1$.

The variances of the estimators are provided by the expressions

$$V\left(\hat{\theta}_A\right) = \frac{\theta_A(1-\theta_A)}{n} + \frac{T(1-P)[PT + (1-P)(1-T)](1 - \theta_A - \theta_B + 2\theta_{AB})}{n(P+T-1)^2},$$

$$V\left(\hat{\theta}_B\right) = \frac{\theta_B(1-\theta_B)}{n} + \frac{P(1-T)[PT + (1-P)(1-T)](1 - \theta_A - \theta_B + 2\theta_{AB})}{n(P+T-1)^2},$$

4.6 Estimation for more than one Sensitive Characteristics

$$V\left(\hat{\theta}_{AB}\right) = \frac{\theta_{AB}(1-\theta_{AB})}{n} - \frac{\theta_{AB}}{n}$$
$$+ \frac{\theta_{AB}\left[P^2T^2 + (1-P)^2(1-T)^2\right] + PT(1-P)(1-T)(1-\theta_A-\theta_B)}{n\left[PT + (1-P)(1-T)\right](P+T-1)^2}.$$

Using the estimators $\hat{\theta}_{AB}$ and $\hat{\theta}_B$, a natural estimator for $\theta_{A|B}$ is given by

$$\hat{\theta}_{A|B} = \frac{\hat{\theta}_{AB}}{\hat{\theta}_B}.$$

Clearly, this estimator is biased and its bias to the first order approximation is given by

$$E\left(\hat{\theta}_{A|B} - \theta_{A|B}\right) \approx \theta_{A|B} \left[\frac{V\left(\hat{\theta}_B\right)}{\theta_B^2} - \frac{\text{Cov}\left(\hat{\theta}_{AB}, \hat{\theta}_B\right)}{\theta_{AB}\theta_B}\right]$$

where

$$\text{Cov}\left(\hat{\theta}_{AB}, \hat{\theta}_B\right) = \frac{\theta_{AB}(1-\theta_B)}{n} + \frac{\theta_{AB}P(1-T)(T-P+1)}{n(P+T-1)^2}$$
$$+ \frac{PT(1-P)(1-T)(P-T+1)(1-\theta_A-\theta_B)}{n\left[PT + (1-P)(1-T)\right](P+T-1)^2}.$$

Finally, the mean squared error to the first order approximation is given by

$$\text{MSE}\left(\hat{\theta}_{A|B}\right) \approx \theta_{AB}^2 \left[\frac{V\left(\hat{\theta}_{AB}\right)}{\theta_{AB}^2} + \frac{V\left(\hat{\theta}_B\right)}{\theta_B^2} - 2\frac{\text{Cov}\left(\hat{\theta}_{AB}, \hat{\theta}_B\right)}{\theta_{AB}\theta_B}\right].$$

It is clear that one can estimate more quantities of interest by using the previously constructed estimators. For example, estimation of the population proportion of people having at least one of the two characteristics can be done via the estimator

$$\hat{\theta}_{A \cup B} = \hat{\theta}_A + \hat{\theta}_B - \hat{\theta}_{AB}.$$

Further details for the Crossed Model can be found in Lee et al. (2013).

4.6.3 Multiple Characteristics

The previously described two methods deal with the problem of estimating two sensitive characteristics at the same time. But in some cases, although rare, there is a need to deal with more than two stigmatizing characteristics. Very few authors have studied this particular problem. See for example Bourke (1981). In this section we will briefly present the more recent approach of Barabesi et al. (2012). Their approach is to extend Franklin's (1989) model to the multiple sensitive items context.

Assume that we are interested in q sensitive items labeled by the first q natural numbers. Let θ_j denote the population proportion of people having the stigmatizing characteristic j, for $j = 1, \ldots, q$. For $m = 1, \ldots, q$ let $G = \{j_1, \ldots, j_m\}$ be a choice of indexes representing m of those stigmatizing items. Clearly, one can have $2^q - 1$ different choices of the set G. Let θ_G be the population proportion of people belonging to the sensitive items of the set G. Let Ψ denote the collection of the sets G arranged in a given order and let $\boldsymbol{\theta} = (\theta_G)_{G \in \Psi}$. The purpose is to estimate the vector $\boldsymbol{\theta}$ using a simple random sample of size n drawn with replacement from the population. Each sampled person i, using a randomization device produces a random variable y_{ji} if he/she has the sensitive characteristic j, otherwise, he/she produces a random variable z_{ji}. We assume that the random variables y_{ji} and z_{ji} are independent for each $i = 1, \ldots, n$ and $j = 1, \ldots, q$ and that for each j, $y_{j1}, \ldots, y_{jn}$ and $z_{j1}, \ldots, z_{jn}$ are respectively independent and identically distributed. Let r_{ji} be the value reported by the i-th sample person regarding the stigmatizing characteristic j. Then r_{ji} can be expressed as

$$r_{ji} = y_{ji} b_{ji} + z_{ji} (1 - b_{ji}) \tag{4.8}$$

where b_{ji} is a Bernoulli random variable with parameter θ_j, assumed to be independent of y_{ji} and z_{ji}. Motivated by (4.8) we define the random variables

$$t_{ji} = \frac{r_{ji} - E(z_{j1})}{E(y_{j1}) - E(z_{j1})}$$

assuming of course that the denominator is not equal to zero. The following estimator is a method of moments estimator for θ_G:

$$\hat{\theta}_G = \frac{1}{n} \sum_{i=1}^{n} T_{Gi}, \ G \in \Psi \tag{4.9}$$

where $T_{Gi} = \prod_{j \in G} t_{ji}$. The estimator is unbiased with variance given by the expression

$$V\left(\hat{\theta}_G\right) = \frac{\phi_G - \theta_G^2}{n} \tag{4.10}$$

where

4.6 Estimation for more than one Sensitive Characteristics

$$\phi_G = E\left[\prod_{j\in G}\left(b_{j1} + \frac{b_{j1}V(y_{j1}) + (1-b_{j1})V(z_{j1})}{(E(y_{j1}) - E(z_{j1}))^2}\right)\right].$$

An unbiased estimator of the variance is provided by

$$\hat{V}\left(\hat{\theta}_G\right) = \frac{1}{n(n-1)}\sum_{i=1}^{n}\left(T_{Gi} - \hat{\theta}_G\right)^2.$$

Let H be another collection of indexes such that $H \in \Psi$ and let $\hat{\theta}_H$ be the estimator of θ_H obtained also by the previous procedure. Then for the purpose of estimating $\theta = (\theta_G)_{G\in\Psi}$ we need the covariance between $\hat{\theta}_G$ and $\hat{\theta}_H$. This covariance can be shown to be

$$Cov\left(\hat{\theta}_G, \hat{\theta}_H\right) = \frac{\phi_{G,H} - \theta_G\theta_H}{n} \quad (4.11)$$

where

$$\phi_{G,H} = E\left[\prod_{j\in G\cap H}\left(b_{j1} + \frac{b_{j1}V(y_{j1}) + (1-b_{j1})V(z_{j1})}{(E(y_{j1}) - E(z_{j1}))^2}\right)\prod_{k\in(G-H)\cup(H-G)}b_{k1}\right].$$

Clearly the covariance is unknown. An unbiased estimator is

$$\hat{Cov}\left(\hat{\theta}_G, \hat{\theta}_H\right) = \frac{\hat{\phi}_{G,H} - \hat{\theta}_G\hat{\theta}_H}{n-1}$$

where

$$\hat{\phi}_{G,H} = \frac{1}{n}\sum_{i=1}^{n}T^2_{(G\cap H)i}T_{((G-H)\cup(H-G))i}.$$

Thus, summarizing, an unbiased estimator of $\theta = (\theta_G)_{G\in\Psi}$ is $\hat{\theta} = \left(\hat{\theta}_G\right)_{G\in\Psi}$ with variance covariance matrix having the diagonal elements given by (4.10) and the off-diagonal elements given by (4.11).

It is possible that the estimators given by (4.9) may assume values outside the parameter space $(0, 1)$ as is often the case with randomized response techniques. The following modified estimator also proposed by Barabesi et al. (2012) offers a solution to the problem. Define the estimator

$$\tilde{\theta}_G = \min\left\{\max\left\{0, \hat{\theta}_G\right\}, 1\right\}.$$

Although this estimator loses some of its nice properties, for example it is no longer unbiased, it is asymptotically equivalent to $\hat{\theta}_G$.

4.7 Some Aspects of Bayesian Approach in Analyzing RR Data

It is well known that Warner (1965) confined his randomized response technique to simple random sampling with replacement alone. Consequently, for estimating $\theta = \left(\sum_{i=1}^{N} y_i\right)/N$ he could write the probability λ of getting a "Yes" response from any person sampled on any one of n draws as

$$\lambda = p\theta + (1-p)(1-\theta)$$

where p is the randomization parameter with $0 < p < 1$, $p \neq 0.5$. Let n_A denote the number of "Yes" responses in the sample. Then n_A follows the binomial distribution with parameters n and λ. So $\hat{\lambda} = n_A/n$ is a maximum likelihood estimator for λ. His conclusion therefore that

$$\hat{\theta} = \frac{1}{2p-1}\left[\frac{n_A}{n} - (1-p)\right]$$

is also the maximum likelihood estimator for θ is now well known to be faulty. This is because the parametric space for θ is the closed interval $[0, 1]$. But depending on the value of p chosen by the investigator, $\hat{\theta}$ may turn out to be negative or may exceed unity. So a correct maximum likelihood estimator for θ is

$$\hat{\theta}_n = \begin{cases} 0 & \text{if } \hat{\theta} < 0 \\ 1 & \text{if } \hat{\theta} > 1 \\ \hat{\theta} & \text{if } 0 < \hat{\theta} < 1. \end{cases}$$

Although $\hat{\theta}$ is unbiased for θ, the same is not true for $\hat{\theta}_n$. This observation is probably at the root of Winkler and Franklin's (1979) desire to go, instead of a maximum likelihood estimator or an unbiased estimator rather for a Bayes estimator for θ. Writing the likelihood for λ obviously as

$$L(\lambda) = \binom{n}{n_A} \lambda^{n_A} (1-\lambda)^{n-n_A}$$

with $\lambda = p\theta + (1-p)(1-\theta)$, Winkler and Franklin (1979) postulated a beta distribution as a prior for θ which is

4.7 Some Aspects of Bayesian Approach in Analyzing RR Data

$$f_B(\theta|\alpha,\beta) = \frac{1}{B(\alpha,\beta)}\theta^{\alpha}(1-\theta)^{\beta-1}, \ \alpha > 0, \ \beta > 0.$$

The likelihood combined with this prior leads to the posterior for θ as

$$g(\theta|n_A,n) \propto \theta^{\alpha-1}(1-\theta)^{\beta-1}[(1-p)+(2p-1)\theta]^{n_A}[p-(2p-1)\theta]^{n-n_A}.$$

This posterior, on expansion of the two terms within the square brackets and simplification, can be written as a linear combination of several beta densities, as expressed by Winkler and Franklin (1979) as follows:

$$g(\theta|n_A,n) = \sum_{t=0}^{n} w_t f_B(\theta|\alpha+t, \beta+n-1), \ 0 \leq \theta \leq 1,$$

where $w_t = w_t^* / \left(\sum_{s=0}^{n} w_s^*\right)$ with

$$w_t^* = \binom{n}{t} \frac{B(\alpha+t, \beta+n-t)}{B(\alpha,\beta)} \sum_{j=0}^{\min\{n_A, t\}} \binom{t}{j}\binom{n-t}{n_A-j} p^{n-t-n_A+2j}(1-p)^{t+n_A-2j}.$$

Opting for a Square Error Loss Function to estimate θ, the choice of an estimator $\hat{\theta}$ is the one which minimizes the posterior expectation $E\left(\hat{\theta}-\theta\right)^2$. This minimizing candidate is the Bayes estimator of θ which is

$$\tilde{\theta}_{\alpha,\beta} = \sum_{t=0}^{n}\left[\frac{w_t(\alpha+t)}{\alpha+\beta+n}\right].$$

Winkler and Franklin (1979) have given approximate numerical calculations to evaluate $\tilde{\theta}_{\alpha,\beta}$.

Pitz (1980) modified this work treating Simmon's randomized response model instead of Warner's, producing similar results.

O'Hagan (1987) derived linear Bayes estimators for θ also based on randomized response data drawn by simple random sampling with replacement confining to Warner's (1965) randomized response model. We omit the details, especially because of the limitations due to simple random sampling with replacement. Of course, he also covered Simmon's model. Pitz (1980) considered an infinite population setup and studied the uniform prior.

Migon and Tachibana (1997) treated Winkler and Franklin's (1979) approach almost verbatim but used the MAPLE code for his approximate computations. He also made use of Tierney and Kadane (1986) to approximately evaluate the posterior mean and posterior variance of θ based on Warner's randomized response data drawn from the population by simple random sampling with replacement.

Unnikrishnan and Kunte (1999) considered a slightly more general randomized response model covering Warner's and Simmon's model with randomized response data based on simple random sampling with replacement and considered Bayes estimation for θ postulating beta priors. This beta-binomial approach leads to computational complications. They demonstrated efficacy of their approach through the Gibbs sampling and MCMC approaches of Metropolis, Rosenbluth, Rosenbluth, Teller, and Teller (1953), Hastings (1970), and Gelfand and Smith (1990).

Bar-Lev, Bobovitch, and Boukai (2003) employed a truncated beta for θ as a conjugate prior in common for several randomized response models applicable to data drawn by simple random sampling with replacement, in common for those due to Warner (1965), Horvitz, Shah, and Simmons (1967) and Greenberg, Abul-Ela, Simmons, and Horvitz (1969), Devore (1977), Fligner, Policello, and Singh (1977), and Mangat and Singh (1990). Their exercise is an extension of Winkler and Franklin's (1979) work.

Kim, Tebbs, and An (2006) used a beta prior for θ to derive for it a Bayes estimator based on data drawn by simple random sampling with replacement derived from an application of Mangat's (1994) model. They used a non-informative prior as well and made a comparative numerical exercise to demonstrate superiority of Bayes' estimators over maximum likelihood estimators.

Barabesi and Marcheselli (2006) made use of data obtained by simple random sampling with replacement from Franklin's (1989) model postulating a beta prior for θ to derive the latter's Bayes estimator. Their theory is along the lines of Winkler and Franklin (1979). But they needed to use the Mathematica package to simplify approximate calculations. Barabesi and Marcheselli (2006) further extended their computational routine with a simulated exercise.

Hussain and Shabbir (2009) considered randomized response data drawn by simple random sampling with replacement to estimate θ employing a usual beta prior but on a randomized response model which is a random modification of Warner's (1965). They use two boxes of cards with compositions of A-marked and A^c-marked cards in different proportions and also prescribing selection of one of them with a given probability and the other with the complimentary probability. They illustrate numerical comparisons among maximum likelihood estimators and Bayes estimators through simulations.

Barabesi and Marcheselli (2010) employ a beta prior for θ but consider Bayes estimation not only of θ but also for the sensitivity level of the stigmatizing attribute by adopting a two-stage randomized response procedure. Their randomized response data are based on simple random sampling with replacement but follow Huang's (2004) model.

For $\sum_{i=1}^{N} y_i$ where y_i is any real number and not necessarily either 0 or 1, to our knowledge no work so far is reported in the literature with a Bayesian approach when randomized response data are gathered. This is no wonder given that the Bayesian literature on estimation based on direct response data is quite scarce except for Basu's (1969) and Ericson's (1969) works.

But in estimating θ from randomized response data, a view propagated in Chaudhuri's (2011) monograph as well as in the present one is that no randomized

4.7 Some Aspects of Bayesian Approach in Analyzing RR Data

response data need to be tied to any specific manner of selecting the sample of individuals from a population $U = (1, \ldots, i, \ldots, N)$. So let us put in a few ideas here about how a Bayes approach may be initiated in the context of randomized response data gathered from a sample by a general selection method when handling qualitative data, specifically as zeros and ones only.

As discussed in the context of providing protection of privacy to respondents (see Chap. 7) let us use the following notation.

Let L_i be the prior probability that y_i is equal to 1. On applying Warner's (1965) randomized response procedure for any person labeled i in a sample s drawn with probability $p(s)$, we have that

$$I_i = \begin{cases} 1 & \text{if the } i\text{-th person's trait matched the card type} \\ 0 & \text{otherwise.} \end{cases}$$

Then for $0 < p < 1$ with $p \neq 0.5$, we may write

$$E_R(I_i) = P(I_i = 1) = py_i + (1-p)(1-y_i) = (1-p) + (2p-1)y_i,$$

$$V_R(I_i) = E_R(I_i)(1 - E_R(I_i)) = p(1-p),$$

$$r_i = \frac{I_i - (1-p)}{2p - 1}$$

with

$$E_R(r_i) = y_i \text{ and } V_R(r_i) = \frac{p(1-p)}{(2p-1)^2}.$$

Let now $L_i(1)$ be the posterior probability that y_i equals 1 given that I_i is equal to 1. Then,

$$L_i(1) = \frac{pL_i}{pL_i + (1-p)(1-L_i)} = \frac{pL_i}{(1-p) + (2p-1)L_i},$$

and it follows that,

$$\frac{1}{L_i(1)} = \frac{1-p}{pL_i} + \frac{2p-1}{p}$$

giving

$$L_i = \frac{1-p}{p} \left(\frac{1}{L_i(1)} - \frac{2p-1}{p} \right)^{-1}.$$

With a somewhat simplified Bayes approach, we may take r_i as an estimator for $L_i(1)$ and hence,

$$\hat{L}_i = \frac{1-p}{p}\left(\frac{1}{r_i} - \frac{2p-1}{p}\right)^{-1} = \alpha\left(\frac{1}{r_i} - \beta\right)^{-1},$$

say, as an estimator for L_i. Then we may employ for the parameter $\Psi = \left(\sum_{i=1}^{N} L_i\right)/N$ the empirical Bayes estimator as

$$\hat{\Psi} = \frac{1}{N}\sum_{i \in s}\frac{\hat{L}_i}{\pi_i},$$

where $\pi_i = \sum_{s \ni i} p(s)$ assumed to be uniformly positive. Again, writing $\pi_{ij} = \sum_{s \ni i,j} p(s)$ and assumed uniformly positive, for the variance

$$V\left(\hat{\Psi}\right) = V_p E_p\left(\hat{\Psi}\right) + E_p V_p\left(\hat{\Psi}\right) \cong \sum_{i}\sum_{j,j>i}(\pi_i \pi_j - \pi_{ij})\left(\frac{L_i}{\pi_i} - \frac{L_j}{\pi_j}\right)^2 + \sum_{i \in s} V_R\left(\hat{L}_i\right)$$

an estimator may be taken as

$$v\left(\hat{\Psi}\right) \cong \sum_{i \in s}\sum_{j \in s, j>i}\left(\frac{\pi_i \pi_j - \pi_{ij}}{\pi_{ij}}\right)\left(\frac{\hat{L}_i}{\pi_i} - \frac{\hat{L}_j}{\pi_j}\right)^2 + \sum_{i \in s} V_R\frac{\left(\hat{L}_i\right)}{\pi_i}.$$

Remark 4.5. Observe that

$$E_R\left(\hat{L}_i\right) \cong \frac{1-p}{p}\left(\frac{1}{L_i(1)} - \frac{2p-1}{p}\right)^{-1} = L_i$$

and

$$V_R\left(\hat{L}_i\right) = \alpha^2 V_R\left(\frac{1}{r_i}\right) \cong \left[\frac{\alpha}{L_i(1)}\right]^2 V_R(r_i).$$

4.8 Further Developments on Randomized Response

There exist, of course, more randomized response devices and techniques in the literature. Some of them are refinements and improvements of others, while a few of them serve a specific purpose. We very briefly mention a few of them.

Alhassan, Ohuchi, and Taguri (1991), Lakshmi and Raghavarao (1992), Chang, Wang, and Huang (2004) take into consideration the probability of dishonest answering in randomized response techniques, given that no one can be sure that participants provide truthful answers.

Hong, Yum, and Lee (1994), Kim and Warde (2004), Christofides (2005a), Kim and Elam (2007) and Lee et al. (2012) consider the case of randomized response when stratification is possible.

Randomized response techniques which allow participants to provide a direct response rather than a randomized response are called optional randomized response techniques. Under this scenario, a participant may consider the issue not sensitive enough, so he/she may choose not to use the randomization device and opt for a direct response. One may consult the works of Mangat (1991), Mangat and Singh (1994), Singh and Joarder (1997b), Arnab (2004), Chaudhuri and Saha (2005), Gupta and Shabbir (2007), Huang (2008), Gupta, Shabbir, and Sehra (2010) and Saha (2011). Optional randomized response is presented in Sect. 5.3.

A recent development combines randomized response with the so called group testing method. The idea behind group testing is that the population can be divided into homogeneous groups and members of the same group behave in the same manner. Thus, a response from one member of the group represents all other members and therefore the sample needed to make inferences can be drastically reduced. In a recent publication, Kim and Heo (2013) combine the two most celebrated randomized response techniques, i.e., Warner's (1965) and the unrelated question model of Greenberg et al. (1969) with group testing. Although there are some benefits in such an approach, the basic assumption of the common behavior of people belonging to the same group should be further studied and validated.

One can mention numerous other extensions and generalizations, but we believe we may not do any harm if we stop at this stage to serve the overall purpose of this book.

References

Alhassan, A.W., Ohuchi, S., Taguri, M. (1991). Randomized response designs considering the probability of dishonest answers. *Journal of the American Statistical Association, 4*, 1–24.
Arnab, R. (2004). Optional randomized response techniques for complex survey designs. *Biometrical Journal, 46*, 114–124.
Bar-Lev, S.K., Bobovitch, E., Boukai, B. (2003). A common conjugate prior structure for several randomized response models. *Test, 12*, 101–113.
Barabesi, L., Franceschi, S., Marcheselli, M. (2012). A randomized response procedure for multiple sensitive questions. *Statistical Papers, 53*, 703–718.
Barabesi, L., & Marcheselli, M. (2006). A practical implementation and Bayesian estimation in Franklin's randomized response procedure. *Communication in Statistics- Simulation and Computation, 35*, 563–573.
Barabesi, L., & Marcheselli, M. (2010). Bayesian estimation of proportion and sensitivity level in randomized response procedures. *Metrika, 72*, 75–88.
Basu, D. (1969). Role of the sufficiency and likelihood principles in sample survey theory. *Sankhya, Series A, 31*, 441–454.
Boruch, R.F. (1972). Relations among statistical methods for assuring confidentiality of social research data. *Social Science Research, 1*, 403–414.
Bourke, P.D. (1981). On the analysis of some multivariate randomized response designs for categorical data. *Journal of Statistical Planning and Inference, 5*, 165–170.

Chang, H.-J., Wang, C.-L., Huang, K.-C. (2004). Using randomized response to estimate the proportion and truthful reporting probability in a dichotomous finite population. *Journal of Applied Statistics, 31,* 565–573.

Chaudhuri, A. (2001a). Using randomized response from a complex survey to estimate a sensitive proportion in a dichotomous finite population. *Journal of Statistical Planning and Inference, 94,* 37–42.

Chaudhuri, A. (2001b). Estimating sensitive proportions from unequal probability samples using randomized responses. *Pakistan Journal of Statistics, 17,* 259–270.

Chaudhuri, A. (2002). Estimating sensitive proportions from randomized responses in unequal probability sampling. *Calcutta Statistical Association Bulletin, 52,* 315–322.

Chaudhuri, A. (2004). Christofides' randomized response technique in complex surveys. *Metrika, 60,* 223–228.

Chaudhuri, A. (2010). *Essentials of survey sampling.* New Delhi: Prentice Hall of India.

Chaudhuri, A. (2011). *Randomized response and indirect questioning techniques in surveys.* Boca Raton: Chapman & Hall, CRC Press, Taylor & Francis Group.

Chaudhuri, A., Adhikary, A.K., Dihidar, S. (2000). Mean square error estimation in multi-stage sampling. *Metrika, 52,* 115–131.

Chaudhuri, A., & Mukerjee, R. (1988). *Randomized response: theory and techniques.* New York: Marcel Dekker.

Chaudhuri, A., & Saha, A. (2005). Optional versus compulsory randomized response techniques in complex surveys. *Journal of Statistical Planning and Inference, 135,* 516–527.

Christofides, T.C. (2003). A generalized randomized response technique. *Metrika, 57,* 195–200.

Christofides, T.C. (2005a). Randomized response in stratified sampling. *Journal of Statistical Planning and Inference, 128,* 303–310.

Christofides, T.C. (2005b). Randomized response technique for two sensitive characteristics at the same time. *Metrika, 62,* 53–63.

Cruyff, M.J.L.F., Bockenholt, U., van der Hout, A., van der Heijden, P.G.M. (2008). Accounting for self-protective responses in randomized response data from social security survey using the zero-inflated Poisson model. *Annals of Applied Statistics, 2,* 316–331.

Dalenius, T., & Vitale, R.A. (1974). A new RR design for estimating the mean of a distribution. *Technical Report,* No 78, Brown University, Providence, RI.

Devore, J.L. (1977). A note on the randomized response technique. *Communications in Statistics - Theory and Methods, 6,* 1525–1529.

Ericson, W.A. (1969). Subjective Bayesian models in sampling finite populations. *Journal of the Royal Statistical Society: Series B, 31,* 195–233.

Fligner, M.A., Policello, G.E., Singh, J. (1977). A comparison of two survey methods with consideration for the level of respondent protection. *Communications in Statistics - Theory and Methods, 6,* 1511–1524.

Fox, J.A., & Tracy, P.E. (1986). *Randomized response: a method for sensitive surveys.* London: Sage.

Franklin, L.A. (1989). A comparison of estimators for randomized response sampling with continuous distributions from a dichotomous population. *Communications in Statistics - Theory and Methods, 18,* 489–505.

Gelfand, A.E., & Smith, A.F.M. (1990). Sampling-based approaches to calculating marginal densities. *Journal of the American Statistical Association, 85,* 398–409.

Godambe, V.P. (1955). A unified theory of sampling from finite populations. *Journal of the Royal Statistical Society: Series B, 17,* 269–278.

Greenberg, B.G., Abul-Ela, A.-L.A., Simmons, W.R., Horvitz, D.G. (1969). The unrelated question RR model: theoretical framework. *Journal of the American Statistical Association, 64,* 520–539.

Gupta, S., & Shabbir, J. (2007). On the estimation of population mean and sensitivity in two-stage optional randomized response model. *Journal of the Indian Society of Agricultural Statistics, 61,* 164–168.

Gupta, S., Shabbir, J., Sehra, S. (2010). Mean and sensitivity estimation in optional randomized response models. *Journal of Statistical Planning and Inference, 140,* 2870–2874.

References

Hastings, W.K. (1970). Monte Carlo sampling methods using Markov Chains and their applications. *Biometrika*, 57, 97–109.

Hong, K., Yum, J., Lee, H. (1994). A stratified randomized response technique. *Korean Journal of Applied Statistics*, 7, 141–147.

Horvitz, D.G., Shah, B.V., Simmons, W.R. (1967). The unrelated question RR model. *Proceedings of the Social Statistics Section of the American Statistical Association* (pp. 65–72). Alexandria, VA: ASA.

Horvitz, D.G., & Thompson, D.J. (1952). A generalization of sampling without replacement from finite universe. *Journal of the American Statistical Association*, 47, 663–685.

Huang, K.-C. (2004). A survey technique for estimating the proportion and sensitivity in a dichotomous finite population. *Statistica Neerlandica*, 58, 75–82.

Huang, K.-C. (2008). Estimation for sensitive characteristics using optional randomized response technique. *Quality and Quantity*, 4, 679–686.

Hussain, Z., & Shabbir, J. (2009). Bayesian estimation of population proportion of a sensitive characteristic using simple beta prior. *Pakistan Journal of Statistics*, 25, 27–35.

Kim, J.-M., & Elam, M.E. (2007). A stratified unrelated question randomized response model. *Statistical Papers*, 48, 215–233.

Kim, J.-M., & Heo, T.-Y. (2013). Randomized response group testing model. *Journal of Statistical Theory and Practice*, 7, 33–48.

Kim, J.-M., Tebbs, J.M., An, S.-W. (2006). Extensions of Mangat's randomized response model. *Journal of Statistical Planning and Inference*, 136, 1554–1567.

Kim, J.-M., & Warde, W.D. (2004). A stratified Warner's randomized response model. *The Journal of Statistical Planning and Inference*, 120, 155–165.

Kuk, A.Y.C. (1990). Asking sensitive questions indirectly. *Biometrika*, 77, 436–438.

Lakshmi, D.V., & Raghavarao, D. (1992). A test for detecting untruthful answering in randomized response procedures. *Journal of Statistical Planning and Inference*, 31, 387–390.

Land, M., Singh, S., Sedory, S.A. (2012). Estimation of a rare sensitive attribute using Poisson distribution. *Statistics*, doi: 10.1080/02331888.2010.524300.

Lee, C.-S., Sedory, S.A., Singh, S. (2013). Estimating at least seven measures of qualitative variables from a single sample using randomized response technique. *Statistics and Probability Letters*, 83, 399–409.

Lee, G.-S., Uhm, D., Kim, J.-M. (2012). Estimation of a rare sensitive attribute in a stratified sample using Poisson distribution. *Statistics*, doi:10.1080/02331888.2011.625503.

Liu, P.T., Chow, L.P., Mosley, W.H. (1975). Use of RR technique with a new randomizing device. *Journal of the American Statistical Association*, 70, 329–332.

Mangat, N.S. (1991). An optional randomized response sampling technique using nonstigmatized attribute. *Statistics*, 51, 595–602.

Mangat, N.S. (1992). Two stage randomized response sampling procedure using unrelated question. *Journal of the Indian Society of Agricultural Statistics*, 44, 82–87.

Mangat, N.S. (1994). An improved randomized response strategy. *Journal of the Royal Statistical Society: Series B*, 56, 93–95.

Mangat, N.S., & Singh, R. (1990). An alternative randomized response procedure. *Biometrika*, 77, 439–442.

Mangat, N.S., Singh, R., Singh, S. (1992). An improved unrelated question randomized response strategy. *Calcutta Statistical Association Bulletin*, 42, 277–281.

Mangat, N.S., & Singh, S. (1994). An optional randomized response sampling technique. *Journal of the Indian Statistical Association*, 32, 71–75.

Metropolis, N., Rosenbluth, A.W., Rosenbluth, M.N., Teller, A.H., Teller, E. (1953). Equations of state calculations by fast computing machines. *Journal of Chemical Physics*, 21, 1087–1092.

Migon, H.S., & Tachibana, V.M. (1997). Bayesian approximations in randomized response model. *Computational Statistics and Data Analysis*, 24, 401–409.

Moshagen, M., & Musch, J. (2011). Surveying multiple sensitive attributes using an extension of the randomized response technique. *International Journal of Public Opinion Research*, doi:10.1093/ijpor/edr034.

O'Hagan, A. (1987). Bayes linear estimators for randomized response models. *Journal of the American Statistical Association, 82*, 580–585.

Pitz, G.F. (1980). Bayesian analysis of random response models. *Psychological Bulletin, 87*, 209–212.

Rao, J.N.K., Hartley, H.O., Cochran, W.G. (1962). On the simple procedure of unequal probability sampling without replacement. *Journal of the Royal Statistical Society: Series B, 24*, 482–491.

Saha, A. (2011). An optional scrambled randomized response technique for practical surveys. *Metrika, 73*, 139–149.

Singh, S., & Grewal, I.S. (2013). Geometric distribution as a randomization device: implemented to the Kuk's model. *International Journal of Contemporary Mathematical Sciences, 8*, 243–248.

Singh, S., & Joarder, A.H. (1997a). Unknown repeated trials in randomized response sampling. *Journal of the Indian Statistical Association, 30*, 109–122.

Singh, S., & Joarder, A.H. (1997b). Optional randomized response technique for sensitive quantitative variable. *Metron, 55*, 151–157.

Tamhane, A.C. (1981). Randomized response techniques for multiple sensitive attributes. *Journal of the American Statistical Association, 76*, 916–923.

Tierney, L., & Kadane, J.B. (1986). Accurate approximations for posterior moments and marginal densities. *Journal of the American Statistical Association, 81*, 82–86.

Unnikrishnan, N.K., & Kunte, S. (1999). Bayesian analysis for randomized response models. *Sankhya Series B, 61*, 422–432.

Walpole, R.E., & Myers, R.H. (1993). *Probability and statistics for engineers and scientists*, 5th edn. Englewood Cliffs, NJ: Prentice-Hall.

Warner, S.L. (1965). Randomized Response: a survey technique for eliminating evasive answer bias. *Journal of the American Statistical Association, 60*, 63–69.

Winkler, R.L., & Franklin, L.A. (1979). Warner's randomized response model: a Bayesian approach. *Journal of the American Statistical Association, 74*, 207–214.

Yates, F., & Grundy, P.M. (1953). Selection without replacement from within strata with probability proportional to size. *Journal of the Royal Statistical Society: Series B, 15*, 253–261.

Chapter 5
Quantitative Issues Bearing Stigma: Parameter Estimation

Abstract A brief outline of the general theory of estimating finite population totals and means based on a sample selected with a suitable sampling design is given. Initially it is assumed that direct responses are available and then the theory is developed in the case when the sensitivity of the data on the quantitative characteristic makes it necessary to implement suitable devices to collect randomized response data. Two different randomized response devices are considered. The theory of estimation is illustrated in case the sample is selected employing the Rao-Hartley-Cochran sampling scheme as well as in the case of a general sampling scheme and when the data are collected using either of the two devices. Techniques which allow for direct responses by participants are presented. Such approaches are based on the idea that some people may consider the item in question not sensitive enough and therefore both options for providing a direct response or a randomized one are available. The main advantage of these optional randomized response techniques is the variance reduction of the produced estimators.

5.1 Introduction

Chaudhuri (2011, pp 91–112) and earlier Chaudhuri and Mukerjee (1988) in their monographs have already given detailed accounts of procedures along with consequences for estimating totals and means of stigmatizing real variables, on gathering, from suitably designed samples randomized responses by dint of various elegant methods. In this compendium we present briefly a few specific results worthy of comprehension and application in practice.

Starting with a population $U = (1, \ldots, i, \ldots, N)$ of a known number of labeled and identifiable units or individual human beings we assume that real variables x, y, z, w, etc. are defined on U. Let $\underline{Y} = (y_1, \ldots, y_i, \ldots, y_N)$, with y_i as the value of y for the i-th unit of U with a total $Y = \sum_{i=1}^{N} y_i$ and similarly $\underline{X}$, $\underline{Z}$, $\underline{W}$ with totals X, Z, W, respectively. A well-developed theory of estimating Y from samples s of U selected with a suitable sampling design p is well known from books and research papers duly cited here and elsewhere. Of course initially we suppose that the values of y_i for $i \in s$ are available as direct responses by dint of surveys. But when the y_i's are not ascertainable because of sensitive issues being involved, randomized responses may have to be procured and analyzed suitably to solve a problem of estimating Y through the randomized responses gathered at hand.

5.2 Theory of Estimating Totals/Means of Stigmatizing Characteristics

For $Y = \sum_{i=1}^{N} y_i$ we need a homogeneous linear unbiased estimator (HLUE) based on a sample s chosen from U with a probability $p(s)$ according to a design p.

Let $(s, y_i \mid i \in s)$ be directly available on surveying the sample s. Let

$$t = \sum_{i \in s} y_i b_{si} = \sum_{i=1}^{N} y_i b_{si} I_{si} = t(s)$$

be such an estimator for Y. Here $I_{si} = 1$ if $i \in s$ and $I_{si} = 0$ otherwise. The b_{si}'s are constants free of $\underline{Y}$. Also $I_{sij} = I_{si} I_{sj}$ for $i \neq j$. Further we need

$$Y = E_p(t) = \sum_s p(s) t(s)$$

so that $\sum_{s \ni i} p(s) b_{si} = 1$ for all i with $p(s) > 0$. Here E_p is the expectation operator with respect to the design p. The variance of t is

$$V_p(t) = E_p(t - Y)^2 = \sum_i C_i y_i^2 + \sum_i \sum_{j, j \neq i} C_{ij} y_i y_j,$$

where

$$C_i = \sum p(s) b_{si}^2 I_{si} - 1, \text{ and } C_{ij} = \sum p(s) b_{si} b_{sj} I_{sij} - 1.$$

An unbiased quadratic estimator for $V_p(t)$ is then

$$v_p(t) = \sum_{i \in s} C_{si} y_i^2 + \sum_{i \in s} \sum_{j \in s, j \neq i} C_{sj} y_i y_j$$

such that

$$\sum_{s \ni i} p(s) C_{si} = C_i, \ \forall \ i \in U$$

5.2 Theory of Estimating Totals/Means of Stigmatizing Characteristics

and

$$\sum_{s \ni i,j} p(s)C_{sij} = C_{ij}, \ \forall \ i, j \in U, \ i \neq j.$$

But our prime concern here is with the situation when direct responses cannot be gathered and the y_i values are too sensitive in nature. Two devices found to be useful in gathering randomized responses relating to quantitative variables that are stigmatizing are reported below.

5.2.1 Device I

A person labeled i is offered two boxes marked A and B, respectively. Cards identical in shape, size, color, dimension, weight, and thickness but bearing numbers $a_1, a_2, \ldots, a_T$ in sufficient numbers are placed in the first box and cards likewise but numbered $b_1, b_2, \ldots, b_M$ are put in the second box. The sampled person i is on request to draw one card independently from each of the boxes, say, bearing a_j and b_k, say, and report the value

$$z_i = a_j y_i + b_k$$

to the investigator without disclosing any of the numbers on the right-hand side. Then,

$$E_R(z_i) = \mu y_i + \gamma, \tag{5.1}$$

where

$$\mu = \frac{1}{T} \sum_{j=1}^{T} a_j \text{ and } \gamma = \frac{1}{M} \sum_{k=1}^{M} b_k.$$

We need to take $\mu \neq 0$. Also,

$$V_R(z_i) = \sigma^2 y_i^2 + \psi^2,$$

where

$$\sigma^2 = \frac{1}{T} \sum_{j=1}^{T} (a_j - \mu)^2, \ \psi^2 = \frac{1}{M} \sum_{k=1}^{M} (b_k - \gamma)^2.$$

From (5.1) it follows that

$$r_i = \frac{z_i - \gamma}{\mu}$$

is such that $E_R(r_i) = y_i$ for all i and

$$V_R(r_i) = \left(\frac{\sigma^2}{\mu^2}\right) y_i^2 + \frac{\psi^2}{\mu^2} = \alpha y_i^2 + \beta, \qquad (5.2)$$

where $\alpha = \sigma^2/\mu^2$ and $\beta = \psi^2/\mu^2$. Employing this randomized response device, it is reasonable to use the revised estimator e for Y with

$$e = e(s) = \sum_{i \in s} r_i b_{si} = \sum_{i=1}^{N} b_{si} I_{si}.$$

Then,

$$E(e) = E_p E_R(e) = E_p(t) = Y,$$

and

$$\begin{aligned}V(e) &= E_p V_R(e) + V_p E_R(e) \\ &= E_p \sum V_i b_{si}^2 + V_p(t) \\ &= \sum V_i (1 + C_i) + \sum y_i^2 C_i + \sum_i \sum_{j, j \neq i} y_i y_j C_{ij}\end{aligned}$$

and also,

$$\begin{aligned}V(e) &= E_R V_p(e) + V_R E_p(e) \\ &= E_R \left(\sum r_i^2 C_i + \sum_i \sum_{j, j \neq i} r_i r_j C_{ij}\right) + V_R \left(\sum_{i=1}^{N} r_i\right) \\ &= \sum y_i^2 C_i + \sum \sum y_i y_j C_{ij} + \sum V_i C_i + \sum V_i,\end{aligned}$$

where $V_i = \alpha y_i^2 + \beta$. We shall write $R = \sum r_i$ and $\underline{R} = (r_1, \ldots, r_i, \ldots, r_N)$. As a consequence,

$$v_1(e) = v_p(t)|_{\underline{Y} = \underline{R}} + \sum_{i \in s} w_i b_{si}$$

and

$$v_2(e) = v_p(t)|_{\underline{Y} = \underline{R}} + \sum_{i \in s} w_i \left(b_{si}^2 - C_{si}\right)$$

5.2 Theory of Estimating Totals/Means of Stigmatizing Characteristics   99

will both unbiasedly estimate $V(e)$. Here

$$w_i = \frac{\alpha r_i^2 + \beta}{1 + \alpha}, \quad E_R(w_i) = V_i, \; i \in U. \tag{5.3}$$

5.2.2 Device II

Suppose a sampled person labeled i is offered a box with a large number of cards of identical shape, dimension, color, thickness, weight, length, and breadth such that a proportion C $(0 < C < 1)$ of them is marked "True" and the remaining of them bearing real values $x_1, x_2, \ldots, x_j, \ldots, x_M$ in proportions $q_1, q_2, \ldots, q_j, \ldots, q_M$ such that $\sum_{j=1}^{M} q_j = 1 - C$. The sampled person i is advised to draw one of the cards and if a card marked "True" is drawn, he/she is to report his/her true value of y, namely y_i. If instead one of the cards marked x_j is drawn, he/she is to report the value x_j and return the card to the box. Denoting the reported value as z_i it follows that

$$E_R(z_i) = C y_i + \sum_{j=1}^{M} q_j x_j.$$

Then,

$$r_i = \frac{1}{C} \left(z_i - \sum_{j=1}^{M} q_j x_j \right)$$

has $E_R(r_i) = y_i$ and since

$$E_R(z_i^2) = C y_i^2 + \sum_{j=1}^{M} q_j x_j^2,$$

then

$$V_i = V_R(r_i) = \frac{1}{C^2} V_R(z_i)$$
$$= \frac{1}{C^2} \left(E_R(z_i^2) - (E_R(z_i))^2 \right)$$
$$= \frac{1}{C^2} \left(C y_i^2 + \sum_{j=1}^{M} q_j x_j^2 - y_i^2 \right)$$
$$= \alpha y_i^2 + \beta y_i + \psi$$

with α, β, and ψ as known numbers in terms of C and x_j, $j = 1, \ldots, M$ and q_j, $j = 1, \ldots, M$. It follows that

$$v_i = \frac{\alpha r_i^2 + \beta r_i + \psi}{1 + \alpha}$$

satisfies

$$E_R(v_i) = V_i, i \in U. \tag{5.4}$$

So, generically, the randomized response data gathered by Device II provide estimators for Y along with variance formulae and unbiased variance estimators formulae similar to the ones yielded by the randomized response data following through Device I.

Chaudhuri (1992) provided the simple formulae (5.1)–(5.4) facilitating unbiased variance estimation in the context of analyzing randomized response data.

For the sake of illustration suppose that from a finite survey population of N persons, a sample of n ($2 < n < N$) persons is selected employing the Rao–Hartley–Cochran's (1962) sampling scheme utilizing known positive normed size-measures P_i such that

$$0 < P_i < 1, i = 1, \ldots, N, \sum_{i=1}^{N} P_i = 1.$$

Starting with Rao, Hartley, and Cochran unbiased estimator

$$t_{RHC} = \sum_n y_i \frac{Q_i}{P_i}$$

with the usual notations, presuming direct responses are available as y_i's to estimate $Y = \sum_{i=1}^{N} y_i$, we have

$$V_P(t_{RHC}) = A \sum_i \sum_{j,j>i} P_i P_j \left(\frac{y_i}{P_i} - \frac{y_j}{P_j} \right)^2,$$

and

$$v_P(t_{RHC}) = B \sum_n \sum_{n'} Q_i Q_{i'} \left(\frac{y_i}{P_i} - \frac{y_{i'}}{P_{i'}} \right)^2$$

where

$$A = \frac{\sum_n N_i^2}{N(N-1)} \text{ and } B = \frac{\sum_n N_i^2 - N}{N^2 - \sum_n N_i^2}.$$

5.2 Theory of Estimating Totals/Means of Stigmatizing Characteristics

Now if the y_i's are stigmatizing and hence unavailable, on employing either of Device I or Device II, unbiased estimators r_i's may be generated for y_i's from randomized response data. Then, we may employ

$$e_{RHC} = \sum_n r_i \frac{Q_i}{P_i}$$

to unbiasedly estimate Y because

$$E(e_{RHC}) = E_p E_R(e_{RHC}) = E_p(t_{RHC}) = Y.$$

Also,

$$V(e_{RHC}) = E_p[V_R(e_{RHC})] + V_p[E_R(e_{RHC})]$$

$$= E_p\left[\sum_n V_i \left(\frac{Q_i}{P_i}\right)^2\right] + V_p(t_{RHC})$$

and again,

$$V(e_{RHC}) = E_R[V_p(e_{RHC})] + V_R[E_p(e_{RHC})]$$

$$= E_R[V_p(t_{RHC})|_{\underline{Y}=\underline{R}}] + V_R\left(\sum_{i=1}^N r_i\right)$$

$$= E_R E_p[v_p(t_{RHC})|_{\underline{Y}=\underline{R}}] + \sum_{i=1}^N V_i.$$

So,

$$v(e_{RHC}) = v_p(t_{RHC})|_{\underline{Y}=\underline{R}} + \sum_n v_i \frac{Q_i}{P_i}$$

is an unbiased estimator for $V(e_{RHC})$.

If, instead, a sample is chosen by a general sampling scheme admitting positive inclusion probabilities π_i, π_{ij} for $i \in U$ and $i \neq j \in U$, then we may start with the Horvitz and Thompson's unbiased estimator

$$t_{HT} = \sum_{i \in s} \frac{y_i}{\pi_i}$$

presuming the y_i's are gathered as direct responses. Then,

$$V_p(t_{HT}) = \sum_i \sum_{j,j>i} (\pi_i \pi_j - \pi_{ij}) \left(\frac{y_i}{\pi_i} - \frac{y_j}{\pi_j} \right)^2$$

and

$$v_p(t_{HT}) = \sum_{i \in s} \sum_{j \in s, j>i} \left(\frac{\pi_i \pi_j - \pi_{ij}}{\pi_{ij}} \right) \left(\frac{y_i}{\pi_i} - \frac{y_j}{\pi_j} \right)^2$$

such that $E_p[v_p(t_{HT})] = V_p(t_{HT})$. But recognizing that the y_i's are stigmatizing and hence not directly available, then employing either Device I or Device II if randomized responses are available and r_i's are derived then, one may employ the derived unbiased estimator

$$e_{HT} = \sum_{i \in s} \frac{r_i}{\pi_i}.$$

Then,

$$V(e_{HT}) = E_R[V_p(e_{HT})] + V_R[E_p(e_{HT})]$$
$$= E_R[E_p v_p(e_{HT})|_{\underline{Y}=\underline{R}}] + V_R\left(\sum_{i=1}^N r_i\right)$$
$$= E_R E_p[v_p(e_{HT})|_{\underline{Y}=\underline{R}}] + \sum_{i=1}^N V_i.$$

Also,

$$V(e_{HT}) = E_p[V_R(e_{HT})] + V_p[E_R(e_{HT})]$$
$$= E_p\left[\sum_{i \in s} \frac{V_i}{\pi_i^2}\right] + V_p(t_{HT}).$$

So,

$$v = v_p(e_{HT})|_{\underline{Y}=\underline{R}} + \sum_{i \in s} \frac{v_i}{\pi_i}$$

provides an unbiased estimator for $V(e_{HT})$.

Those who are interested to gather how the theory generally applicable to direct response-based sampling design regarding estimation can be extended to the randomized response situation will do well to peruse Chaudhuri (2011).

5.3 Optional Randomized Response

In many cases, a characteristic considered sensitive by some people may be considered nonsensitive by others. For example, homosexuality and sexual orientation in general may be considered sensitive or nonsensitive depending on the personal approach and beliefs of the people asked. A sampled person may choose to provide a direct response instead of a randomized one. Thus the concept of optional randomized response has emerged where a (random) subsample of the respondents provide direct responses and the remaining respondents provide randomized responses via the use of a randomization device. Optional randomized response first introduced by Chaudhuri and Mukerjee (1985, 1988) has recently attracted a lot of attention.

Before we present the optional randomized response methodology and approach, we present the Eichhorn and Hayre (1983) scrambling procedure, on which some of the most recent optional randomized response techniques are based.

Eichhorn and Hayre (1983) use the approach of multiplicative scrambling to produce a randomized response technique. In their approach, let y be the random variable denoting the true (stigmatizing) response. Let also s denote a scrambling variable which is independent of y, with known mean μ_s ($\mu_s \neq 0$) and variance σ_s^2. Each respondent masks his/her true y with the use of the scrambling variable s by reporting the value $z = ys/\mu_s$. For practical purposes, the scrambling variable can be chosen by the researcher so that $\mu_s = 1$ and therefore we avoid the unnecessary step of asking the sampled people to multiply by s and then divide by μ_s.

It is clear that $E(z) = E(y)$. Thus, a natural and immediate estimator $\hat{\mu}_y$ of μ_y is

$$\hat{\mu}_y \equiv \bar{z} = \frac{1}{n} \sum_{i=1}^{n} z_i$$

assuming that $z_1, \ldots, z_n$ are the responses of a random sample of size n drawn with replacement from the population. The variance of the estimator is given by

$$V(\hat{\mu}_y) = \frac{\sigma_z^2}{n} = \frac{1}{n}\left[\sigma_y^2 + \frac{\sigma_s^2}{\mu_s^2}\left(\sigma_y^2 + \mu_y^2\right)\right]. \tag{5.5}$$

Obviously, an unbiased estimator for the variance in (5.5) is given by using the sample variance s_z^2 as an estimator of σ_z^2 and therefore we obtain the estimator

$$\hat{V}(\hat{\mu}_y) = \frac{s_z^2}{n} = \frac{1}{n(n-1)} \sum_{i=1}^{n} (z_i - \bar{z})^2.$$

Gupta, Gupta, and Singh (2002) modified the approach of Eichhorn and Hayre (1983) to cover the case where some of the participants give direct responses and the rest provide randomized responses. The proportion of people who consider the question sensitive enough so that they choose to give a randomized response is called the sensitivity level of the question. Each sampled person gives either a direct response or a scrambled response, without disclosing whether the response is a direct response or not. Let w denote the sensitivity level of the question. Then a participant's response z is:

$$z = \begin{cases} y & \text{with probability } 1-w \\ ys & \text{with probability } w, \end{cases}$$

where y is the true value of the sensitive characteristic and s is the scrambling variable. As in the Eichhorn and Hayre (1983) approach, the scrambling variable s is assumed to be independent of the sensitive variable y with known mean μ_s ($\mu_s \neq 0$) and variance σ_s^2. It is trivial to see that $E(z) = E(y)$ and thus it is natural again to use as an estimator $\hat{\mu}_y$ of μ_y the sample average $\bar{z} = \left(\sum_{i=1}^n z_i\right)/n$ of the values $z_1, \ldots, z_n$ of a random sample of size n drawn with replacement from the population. The variance of the estimator is provided by the expression

$$V(\hat{\mu}_y) = \frac{\sigma_z^2}{n} = \frac{1}{n}\left[\sigma_y^2 + w\frac{\sigma_s^2}{\mu_s^2}\left(\sigma_y^2 + \mu_y^2\right)\right]. \tag{5.6}$$

An obvious unbiased estimator of the variance is

$$\hat{V}(\hat{\mu}_y) = \frac{s_z^2}{n} = \frac{1}{n(n-1)}\sum_{i=1}^n (z_i - \bar{z})^2.$$

By examining (5.5) and (5.6) we conclude that the optional randomized response approach leads to a smaller variance of the estimator.

An important issue in optional randomized response is the estimation of the unknown sensitivity level of the question. Observe that the response z provided can alternatively be written as

$$z = xys^x, \tag{5.7}$$

where x is a Bernoulli random variable with parameter w. From (5.7) one easily obtains that

$$w = \frac{E(lnz) - E(lny)}{E(lns)}.$$

In the above equation, the quantity $E(lns)$ is clearly known and $E(lnz)$ can be estimated by the quantity $\left(\sum_{i=1}^n lnz_i\right)/n$. Thus, as soon as an estimator of $E(lny)$ is available, we can estimate the sensitivity level of the question. Using a first order Taylor approximation for lny, we finally get the following estimator

5.3 Optional Randomized Response

$$\hat{w} = \frac{\frac{1}{n}\sum_{i=1}^{n} \ln z_i - \ln \bar{z}}{E(\ln s)}. \tag{5.8}$$

The above estimator in (5.8) is clearly biased. In addition, its variance is not easy to calculate. To overcome these difficulties, modified procedures have been suggested by Huang (2010) and Gupta, Shabbir, and Sehra (2010). Both approaches require two samples but they differ in the sense that one uses multiplicative and additive scrambling and the other additive scrambling only.

5.3.1 The Approach of Huang (2010)

Suppose that we have two independent simple random samples of sizes n_1 and n_2 drawn with replacement from the population. Each sampled person from the k-th sample, $k = 1, 2$, is provided with two randomization devices. With the use of the devices in the absence of the interviewer, the participant generates two positive random observations s_k and t_k from known distributions. Then the participant reports a value which is either one of the following two values:

(i) The true value of y
(ii) The masked value $s_k y + t_k$.

Assume that $\mu_{s_1}, \mu_{s_2}, \mu_{t_1}, \mu_{t_2}$ are the known means with $\mu_{s_1} = \mu_{s_2} = 1$, $\mu_{t_1} \neq \mu_{t_2}$ and $\sigma_{s_1}^2, \sigma_{s_2}^2, \sigma_{t_1}^2, \sigma_{t_2}^2$ the known variances of the random observations s_1, s_2, t_1, t_2. Clearly the response provided by a person from the k-th sample, $k = 1, 2$, is

$$z_k = (1 - x)y + x(s_k y + t_k), \tag{5.9}$$

where x is a Bernoulli random variable with parameter w and w is the sensitivity level of the question. The random variable x is assumed to be independent from all other variables involved. By applying the expectation operation to (5.9) we have that for $k = 1, 2$,

$$\begin{aligned} E(z_k) &= (1 - E(x)) E(y) + E(x) (E(s_k) E(y) + E(t_k)) \\ &= (1 - w)\mu_y + w(\mu_y + \mu_{t_k}) \\ &= \mu_y + w\mu_{t_k}. \end{aligned} \tag{5.10}$$

From the two equations given in (5.10) it follows that

$$\mu_y = \frac{\mu_{t_1} E(z_2) - \mu_{t_2} E(z_1)}{\mu_{t_1} - \mu_{t_2}}$$

and

$$w = \frac{E(z_1) - E(z_2)}{\mu_{t_1} - \mu_{t_2}}.$$

Assuming that $z_{k1}, z_{k2}, \ldots, z_{kn_k}$ are the responses provided by the participants of the k-th sample, the previous two equations suggest that unbiased estimators of μ_y and w are given by

$$\hat{\mu}_y = \frac{\mu_{t_1}\bar{z}_2 - \mu_{t_2}\bar{z}_1}{\mu_{t_1} - \mu_{t_2}}$$

and

$$\hat{w} = \frac{\bar{z}_1 - \bar{z}_2}{\mu_{t_1} - \mu_{t_2}},$$

where $\bar{z}_k = \left(\sum_{i=1}^{n_k} z_{ki}\right)/n_k$ is the k-th sample average of the responses for $k = 1, 2$. The variance expressions for the two estimators are

$$V(\hat{\mu}_y) = \frac{1}{(\mu_{t_1} - \mu_{t_2})^2} \left(\mu_{t_2}^2 \frac{\sigma_{z_1}^2}{n_1} + \mu_{t_1}^2 \frac{\sigma_{z_2}^2}{n_2} \right),$$

where

$$\sigma_{z_k}^2 = \sigma_y^2 + w\sigma_{s_k}^2 \left(\sigma_y^2 + \mu_y^2 \right) + w\sigma_{t_k}^2 + w(1-w)\mu_{t_k}^2, \quad k = 1, 2, \quad (5.11)$$

and

$$V(\hat{w}) = \frac{1}{(\mu_{t_1} - \mu_{t_2})^2} \left(\frac{\sigma_{z_1}^2}{n_1} + \frac{\sigma_{z_2}^2}{n_2} \right).$$

The above variances are unknown. Obviously, unbiased estimators of the variances are given by

$$\hat{V}(\hat{\mu}_y) = \frac{1}{(\mu_{t_1} - \mu_{t_2})^2} \left(\mu_{t_2}^2 \frac{s_{z_1}^2}{n_1} + \mu_{t_1}^2 \frac{s_{z_2}^2}{n_2} \right)$$

and

$$\hat{V}(\hat{w}) = \frac{1}{(\mu_{t_1} - \mu_{t_2})^2} \left(\frac{s_{z_1}^2}{n_1} + \frac{s_{z_2}^2}{n_2} \right),$$

5.3 Optional Randomized Response

respectively, where

$$s_{z_k}^2 = \frac{1}{n_k - 1} \sum_{i=1}^{n_k} (z_{ki} - \bar{z}_k)^2, \quad k = 1, 2.$$

A relevant issue is the estimation of the variance σ_y^2 of the sensitive characteristic y. From the two equations given by (5.11), and assuming that $\sigma_{s_1}^2 \neq \sigma_{s_2}^2$, we have that

$$\sigma_y^2 = \frac{\sigma_{s_2}^2 \sigma_{z_1}^2 - \sigma_{s_1}^2 \sigma_{z_2}^2 - w \left(\sigma_{s_2}^2 \sigma_{t_1}^2 - \sigma_{s_1}^2 \sigma_{t_2}^2 \right) - w(1-w) \left(\sigma_{s_2}^2 \mu_{t_1}^2 - \sigma_{s_1}^2 \mu_{t_2}^2 \right)}{\sigma_{s_2}^2 - \sigma_{s_1}^2},$$

which suggests the following estimator

$$\hat{\sigma}_y^2 = \frac{\sigma_{s_2}^2 \sigma_{z_1}^2 - \sigma_{s_1}^2 \sigma_{z_2}^2 - \hat{w} \left(\sigma_{s_2}^2 \sigma_{t_1}^2 - \sigma_{s_1}^2 \sigma_{t_2}^2 \right) - \left[\hat{w}(1-\hat{w}) + \hat{V}(\hat{w}) \right] \left(\sigma_{s_2}^2 \mu_{t_1}^2 - \sigma_{s_1}^2 \mu_{t_2}^2 \right)}{\sigma_{s_2}^2 - \sigma_{s_1}^2}.$$

The above estimator can be shown to be unbiased, based on the observation that the quantity $\hat{w}(1 - \hat{w}) + \hat{V}(\hat{w})$ is an unbiased estimator of $w(1 - w)$.

5.3.2 The Approach of Gupta, Shabbir and Sehra (2010)

In this method, again we assume that we have two independent simple random samples of sizes n_1 and n_2 drawn with replacement from the population. Each sampled person from the k-th sample, $k = 1, 2$ is asked to do one of the following two things, the first with probability p and the second with the complementary probability $1 - p$:

(a) To provide the true value of the stigmatizing variable y
(b) To either provide the true value of y or the masked value $y + s_k$,

where s_1, s_2 are independent scrambling variables which are also independent from y. Assuming as before that w is the sensitivity level of the stigmatizing item, then the response z_k provided by a respondent from the k-th sample is:

$$z_k = \begin{cases} y & \text{with probability } p + (1-p)(1-w) \\ y + s_k & \text{with probability } (1-p)w. \end{cases}$$

Alternatively, z_k can be expressed as

$$z_k = xy + (1-x)\left[y(1-r) + (y + s_k)r \right]$$
$$= y + (1-x)r s_k, \tag{5.12}$$

where x and r are independent Bernoulli random variables (and independent from all other variables involved) with parameters p and w, respectively.

Assume that μ_{s_1}, μ_{s_2} with $\mu_{s_1} \neq \mu_{s_2}$ denote the means and $\sigma_{s_1}^2, \sigma_{s_2}^2$ the variances of the scrambling variables s_1 and s_2. Then from (5.12) we have that

$$E(z_k) = \mu_y + \mu_{s_k} w(1-p), \quad k = 1, 2. \tag{5.13}$$

Solving the system of the two equations in (5.13) for μ_y and w we obtain that

$$\mu_y = \frac{\mu_{s_1} E(z_2) - \mu_{s_2} E(z_1)}{\mu_{s_1} - \mu_{s_2}}$$

and

$$w = \frac{E(z_1) - E(z_2)}{(1-p)(\mu_{s_1} - \mu_{s_2})}.$$

Assuming that $z_{k1}, z_{k2}, \ldots, z_{kn_k}$ are the responses provided by the participants of the k-th sample, the previous two expressions suggest as unbiased estimators of μ_y and the sensitivity level w the quantities

$$\hat{\mu}_y = \frac{\mu_{s_1} \bar{z}_2 - \mu_{s_2} \bar{z}_1}{\mu_{s_1} - \mu_{s_2}}$$

and

$$\hat{w} = \frac{\bar{z}_1 - \bar{z}_2}{(1-p)(\mu_{s_1} - \mu_{s_2})},$$

where $\bar{z}_k = \left(\sum_{i=1}^{n_k} z_{ki}\right)/n_k$ is the k-th sample average of the responses for $k = 1, 2$. The variances of the estimators are given by

$$V(\hat{\mu}_y) = \frac{1}{(\mu_{s_1} - \mu_{s_2})^2} \left(\mu_{s_2}^2 \frac{\sigma_{z_1}^2}{n_1} + \mu_{s_1}^2 \frac{\sigma_{z_2}^2}{n_2} \right)$$

and

$$V(\hat{w}) = \frac{1}{(1-p)^2 (\mu_{t_1} - \mu_{t_2})^2} \left(\frac{\sigma_{z_1}^2}{n_1} + \frac{\sigma_{z_2}^2}{n_2} \right).$$

As in the case of the approach of Huang (2010), unbiased estimators of the variances are given by

$$\hat{V}(\hat{\mu}_y) = \frac{1}{(\mu_{s_1} - \mu_{s_2})^2} \left(\mu_{s_2}^2 \frac{s_{z_1}^2}{n_1} + \mu_{s_1}^2 \frac{s_{z_2}^2}{n_2} \right)$$

and

$$\hat{V}(\hat{w}) = \frac{1}{(1-p)^2(\mu_{t_1}-\mu_{t_2})^2}\left(\frac{s_{z_1}^2}{n_1}+\frac{s_{z_2}^2}{n_2}\right).$$

A relevant issue is the estimation of the variance σ_y^2 of the stigmatizing variable y. From (5.12) we have that

$$\begin{aligned}\sigma_{z_k}^2 &= \sigma_y^2 + Var\left((1-x)rs_k\right)\\ &= \sigma_y^2 + E\left((1-x)^2 r^2 s_k^2\right) - (E\left((1-x)rs_k\right))^2\\ &= \sigma_y^2 + (1-p)w\left(\sigma_{s_k}^2 + \mu_{s_k}^2\right) - (1-p)^2 w^2 \mu_{s_k}^2, \ k=1,2.\end{aligned}$$

Combining these two equations, one can show that

$$\sigma_y^2 = \frac{\mu_{s_1}^2 \sigma_{z_2}^2 - \mu_{s_2}^2 \sigma_{z_1}^2 - w(1-p)\left(\mu_{s_1}^2 \sigma_{s_2}^2 - \mu_{s_2}^2 \sigma_{s_1}^2\right)}{\mu_{s_1}^2 - \mu_{s_2}^2}.$$

Obviously, the above equation points out that an unbiased estimator of σ_y^2 is the estimator

$$\hat{\sigma}_y^2 = \frac{\mu_{s_1}^2 s_{z_2}^2 - \mu_{s_2}^2 s_{z_1}^2 - \hat{w}(1-p)\left(\mu_{s_1}^2 \sigma_{s_2}^2 - \mu_{s_2}^2 \sigma_{s_1}^2\right)}{\mu_{s_1}^2 - \mu_{s_2}^2},$$

where, as before, $s_{z_k}^2$ denotes the usual unbiased estimator of $\sigma_{z_k}^2$, for $k=1,2$.

5.3.3 Optional Randomized Response for Complex Sampling Designs

The approaches so far presented are for the case of drawing a simple random sample from the population with replacement. However, in many cases more complex sampling strategies are implemented. Arnab (2004) presented a strategy which deals with optional randomized response for complex survey designs. His approach covers both qualitative and quantitative stigmatizing characteristics. In this subsection we briefly present Arnab's (2004) approach.

Assume that from a finite population $U = (1,\ldots,i,\ldots,N)$ of size N a sample s of size n is drawn using a sampling design p. Assume further that π_i and π_{ij}, i.e., the first and second order inclusion probabilities are positive. The purpose is to estimate μ_y, the population mean of the stigmatizing characteristic y. For the i-th respondent, let y_i denote the true value of the stigmatizing characteristic. Each one of the people selected in the sample has the option to provide the true value

y_i if he/she feels that the characteristics is not stigmatizing enough, or provide a randomized response r_i. Let us denote by G the subset of people in the sample opting to provide a randomized response, while by G^c is denoted the subset of the sample who choose to provide the true value of the characteristic applicable to them. Let E_R, V_R, and C_R denote the expectation, variance, and covariance operator, respectively, with respect to the randomized response device. Assume that the randomized response procedure is such that

$$E_R(r_i) = y_i, \; V_R(r_i) = \sigma_i^2, \; C_R(r_i, r_j) = 0, \; i \neq j.$$

Define the following indicator function

$$I_i = \begin{cases} 1 \text{ if } i \in G^c \\ 0 \text{ if } i \in G. \end{cases}$$

Furthermore define the estimator

$$t = \sum_{i \in s} b_{si} \tilde{r}_i, \tag{5.14}$$

where $\tilde{r}_i = I_i y_i + (1 - I_i) r_i$ and b_{si} are constants such that

$$\sum_{s \ni i} b_{si} p(s) = \frac{1}{N}.$$

Then the following theorem of Arnab (2004) shows unbiasedness for t and gives its variance.

Theorem 5.1. *The quantity t is an unbiased estimator of μ_y with variance*

$$V(t) = \sum_{i=1}^{N} (\alpha_i - 1) y_i^2 + \sum_{i=1}^{N} \sum_{j=1, j \neq i}^{N} (\alpha_{ij} - 1) y_i y_j + \sum_{i \in G} \alpha_i \sigma_i^2, \tag{5.15}$$

where

$$\alpha_i = \sum_{s \ni i} b_{si}^2 p(s) \text{ and } \alpha_{ij} = \sum_{s \ni i,j} b_{si} b_{sj} p(s). \tag{5.16}$$

Obviously the variance of t is unknown. Arnab (2004) provides for the variance the following unbiased estimator

$$\hat{V}(t) = \sum_{i \in s} d_{si} \tilde{r}_i^2 + \sum_{i \in s} \sum_{j \in s, j \neq i} d_{sij} \tilde{r}_i \tilde{r}_j + \sum_{i \in G_s} d_{si}^* \hat{\sigma}_i^2, \tag{5.17}$$

5.3 Optional Randomized Response

where d_{si}, d_{sij}, and d_{si}^* are quantities independent of the $\tilde{r}_i$'s satisfying the conditions

$$\sum_{s \ni i} d_{si} p(s) = \alpha_i - 1, \quad \sum_{s \ni i} d_{sij} p(s) = \alpha_{ij} - 1, \quad \sum_{s \ni i} d_{si}^* p(s) = 1,$$

$\hat{\sigma}_i^2$ is an unbiased estimator of σ_i^2 and G_s is the subset of respondents providing a randomized response.

As pointed out by Arnab (2004) the quantities d_{si}, d_{sij}, and d_{si}^* can be chosen in various ways with one possible choice to be

$$d_{si} = \frac{1 - \alpha_i}{\pi_i}, \quad d_{sij} = \frac{1 - \alpha_{ij}}{\pi_{ij}}, \quad \text{and} \quad d_{si}^* = \frac{1}{\pi_i}.$$

In equation (5.14), by choosing $b_{si} = 1/(N\pi_i)$ we obtain the Horvitz–Thompson estimator

$$t_{HT} = \frac{1}{N} \sum_{i \in s} \frac{\tilde{r}_i}{\pi_i}.$$

For this choice of the b_{si}'s by (5.16), we have that

$$\alpha_i = \frac{1}{N^2 \pi_i} \quad \text{and} \quad \alpha_{ij} = \frac{1}{N^2 \pi_{ij}}.$$

From (5.15) the variance of the estimator is

$$V(t_{HT}) = \frac{1}{N^2} \left[\sum_{i=1}^{N} \sum_{j=1, j>i}^{N} (\pi_i \pi_j - \pi_{ij}) \left(\frac{y_i}{\pi_i} - \frac{y_j}{\pi_j} \right)^2 + \sum_{i \in G} \frac{\sigma_i^2}{\pi_i} \right],$$

and from (5.17) the estimated variance is given as

$$\hat{V}(t_{HT}) = \frac{1}{N^2} \left[\sum_{i \in s} \sum_{j \in s, j>i} \left(\frac{\pi_i \pi_j - \pi_{ij}}{\pi_{ij}} \right) \left(\frac{\tilde{r}_i}{\pi_i} - \frac{\tilde{r}_j}{\pi_j} \right)^2 + \sum_{i \in G_s} \frac{\hat{\sigma}_i^2}{\pi_i} \right].$$

For the SRSWOR design, obviously

$$\pi_i = \frac{n}{N} \quad \text{and} \quad \pi_{ij} = \frac{n(n-1)}{N(N-1)}$$

leading to

$$t = \frac{1}{n} \sum_{i \in s} \tilde{r}_i$$

as our estimator with variance

$$V(t) = \frac{N-n}{nN}S_y^2 + \frac{1}{nN}\sum_{i \in G}\sigma_i^2$$

and estimated variance

$$\hat{V}(t) = \frac{N-n}{nN}s_r^2 + \frac{1}{nN}\sum_{i \in G_s}\hat{\sigma}_i^2,$$

where

$$S_y^2 = \frac{1}{N-1}\sum_{i=1}^N (y_i - \mu_y)^2 \text{ and } s_r^2 = \frac{1}{n-1}\sum_{i \in s}(\tilde{r}_i - \bar{\tilde{r}})^2$$

with $\bar{\tilde{r}}$ denoting the sample average of $\tilde{r}_1, \ldots, \tilde{r}_n$.

Remark 5.1. The form the estimator takes in (5.14) and its associated variance and estimated variance for various other sampling designs can be found in Arnab (2004).

Chaudhuri and Saha (2005), Pal (2008) and Chaudhuri and Dihidar (2009) have given further details concerning this topic on optional randomized response covering both qualitative and quantitative variables. These are briefly narrated also by Chaudhuri (2011, chapters 5 and 9).

References

Arnab, R. (2004). Optional randomized response techniques for complex survey designs. *Biometrical Journal, 46*, 114–124.

Chaudhuri, A. (1992). Randomized response: Estimating mean square errors of linear estimators and finding optimal unbiased strategies. *Metrika, 39*, 341–357.

Chaudhuri, A. (2011). *Randomized response and indirect questioning techniques in surveys*. Boca Raton: Chapman & Hall, CRC Press, Taylor & Francis Group.

Chaudhuri, A., & Dihidar, K. (2009). Estimating means of stigmatizing qualitative and quantitative variables from discretionary responses randomized or direct. *Sankhya Series B, 71*, 123–136.

Chaudhuri, A., & Mukerjee, R. (1985). Optionally randomized response techniques. *Calcutta Statistical Association Bulletin, 34*, 225–229.

Chaudhuri, A., & Mukerjee, R. (1988). *Randomized response: theory and techniques*. New York: Marcel Dekker.

Chaudhuri, A., & Saha, A. (2005). Optional versus compulsory randomized response techniques in complex surveys. *Journal of Statistical Planning and Inference, 135*, 516–527.

Eichhorn, B.H., & Hayre, L.S. (1983). Scrambled randomized response methods for obtaining quantitative data. *Journal of Statistical Planning and Inference, 7*, 306–316.

Gupta, S., Gupta, B., Singh, S. (2002). Estimation of sensitivity level of personal interview survey question. *Journal of Statistical Planning and Inference, 100*, 239–247.

References

Gupta, S., Shabbir, J., Sehra, S. (2010). Mean and sensitivity estimation in optional randomized response models. *Journal of Statistical Planning and Inference, 140*, 2870–2874.

Huang, K.-C. (2010). Unbiased estimators of mean, variance and sensitivity level for quantitative characteristics in finite population sampling. *Metrika, 71*, 341–352.

Pal, S. (2008). Unbiasedly estimating the total of a stigmatizing variable from a complex survey on permitting options for direct or randomized responses. *Statistical Papers, 49*, 157–164.

Rao, J.N.K., Hartley, H.O., Cochran, W.G. (1962). On the simple procedure of unequal probability sampling without replacement. *Journal of the Royal Statistical Society: Series B, 24*, 482–491.

Chapter 6
Indirect Techniques as Alternatives to Randomized Response

Abstract Numerous randomized response techniques have been developed to handle the case of stigmatizing characteristics. Warner's (1965) pioneering technique was just the beginning. One of the main disadvantages of randomized response techniques is the fact that participants often are very skeptical about the whole process because, either they do not understand it or because they feel that their privacy is not really protected. In addition, in cases where a randomization device is being used, people think of randomized response as a trick, or as a process which is not really a serious scientific method. Because of these and other drawbacks, for example the fact that randomized response very rarely can be incorporated into survey questionnaires, other alternative methods have been devised. In this chapter, five of those techniques and their variations are presented along with the relevant theory. The most popular one, the Item Count Technique is discussed first, and various versions of it are given. Another technique included in this chapter is the Nominative Technique, which, as explained, can be thought of as an application of network sampling. The Three-Card Method, a simple and easily understood technique is also discussed in brief with theoretical details omitted. A special treatment is given to the recently developed class of Non-Randomized Models. Those are techniques which do not use any device. However, this does not mean that no randomizations are taking place. The last section of the chapter is devoted to the so-called Negative Surveys. Those are surveys where questions are phrased in a negative way so that all but one of the possible answers are true for each and everyone one of the participants.

6.1 Introduction

Many researchers, mainly from the social sciences seem to dislike randomized response for various reasons. One of them is related to the fact that questionnaires, a crucial instrument for obtaining multiple information on various aspects in social research, very rarely can be used in combination with a randomization device.

Thus, instead they prefer alternative methods, one of which, the most popular one, is the so-called Item Count Technique. A group of people is presented with a list of non-stigmatizing statements. Each one of the members of the group, without revealing which ones, is asked to say only how many of those statements apply to him/her. A second group of people, independent from the first one is presented with a list which, in addition to the non-stigmatizing statements, a statement related to a sensitive item is included. Again, each one of the members of the group is asked to only indicate the number of statements applicable to him/her. By comparing the responses of the two groups, one can estimate the prevalence of the stigmatizing characteristic.

Another alternative to randomized response is the "Nominative Technique." In this method, each of the sampled persons is asked to indicate, i.e., nominate as many of his/her acquaintances have the stigmatizing characteristic. For example, he/she may be asked to say how many people he/she is aware of making illegal drug use.

The third alternative is the so-called the "Three-Card Method" introduced by Droitcour, Larson, and Scheuren (2001). This technique requires three independent samples. Various answer categories are grouped in three boxes. The answer categories are arranged in such a way that the stigmatizing item is in one of the boxes but along with other innocuous items. Each respondent is asked to indicate the box number applicable to him/her.

A newly developed methodology, avoids the use of any randomization device to produce a response from a participant from which it is not possible to infer whether the specific person has the stigmatizing characteristic or not. Although such techniques could be called device free randomized response models, they are known as Non Randomized Models. The term used is somewhat misleading and gives the impression that no randomization takes place. However, the randomization is implicit in those procedures.

A final method to be presented in this chapter deals with questionnaires with "negative questions," i.e., questions with multiple answers, all of which are applicable to a participant except one. The participant is requested to choose one of those answers and report it to the interviewer. The term "negative question" will be fully justified in Sect. 6.6.

Various findings indicate that so far, none of the above methods is trouble free. Various authors and practitioners are offering improvements and modifications to overcome faults and difficulties mainly having to do with the protection of privacy and the cooperation of the participants. In addition, unlike the case of randomized response techniques where the issue of estimating quantitative characteristics has been substantially covered, in the methods that are presented in this chapter, the issue of quantitative characteristics has not really been addressed. As it can be easily understood, it is really not feasible to use the nominative technique or the three-card method for such an estimation. However, there might be a modification of the methodology governing the item count technique which will allow its implementation for estimating quantitative sensitive characteristics. Such a modification is presented in Sect. 6.2.3.

6.2 The Item Count Technique

The Item Count Technique (or List Experiments or Block Total Response or Unmatched Count Technique) originally introduced by Raghavarao and Federer (1979), Miller (1984) and Miller, Cisin, and Harrel (1986), is popular among social researchers. It can be easily understood by participants and it can be incorporated in large-scale surveys in which the instrument of collecting information is a structured questionnaire. In the original version of this technique, two independent samples from the population are required. Each one of the participants of the first group is given a list containing say, G innocuous items and he/she is asked to report to the investigator the number of those items applicable to him/her, without revealing which ones apply. Each one of the people in the second sample is presented with a list containing $G + 1$ items, i.e., the same G innocuous items presented to the first sample and, one item, which is the sensitive one. The difference between the sample mean number of items reported by the two groups is an estimate of the proportion of people in the population bearing the stigmatizing characteristic. The parameter G should be chosen wisely. Very small values are likely to create problems of confidentiality and very large ones inflate the variance of the estimator and in addition are likely to create problems of cooperation and difficulties with time and resource constraints.

6.2.1 Revised Version of the Item Count Technique

The method as described above, has a serious disadvantage which is related to the protection of privacy. In case all $G + 1$ items are applicable (or none) to a respondent of the second sample, then his/her response reveals his/her status concerning the stigmatizing characteristic and thus the issue of privacy protection arises. To remedy this problem Chaudhuri and Christofides (2007) proposed a modification of the technique, which we now present.

Let θ be the unknown proportion of people having the sensitive characteristic A in a population of N persons. Let F be an innocuous characteristic whose prevalence in the population is known, say θ_F and assume that it is independent of A. A simple random sample of size n_1 drawn with replacement from the population is given a questionnaire consisting of G innocuous items-statements and of the $(G + 1)$-st item which is the following:

I have characteristic A or characteristic F.

Each respondent reports just the number of statements which are applicable to him/her, i.e., one of the numbers $0, 1, \ldots, G, G + 1$. In no way, a participant should disclose which statements are applicable to him/her. Observe that the statement related to the sensitive characteristic is applicable to a person if that person has the stigmatizing characteristic A or the innocuous characteristic F or both. This should be clearly explained to the participants as soon as the questionnaire is given to them.

A second simple random sample of size n_2 drawn with replacement from the population, independent of the first, is given a questionnaire consisting of the same G innocuous statements as the first questionnaire, and in addition a $(G+1)$-st statement which is the following:

I do not have characteristic A or I do not have characteristic F.

Again, each participant is to report the number of items applicable to him/her. Observe that the item related to characteristic A is applicable to a person if that person does not have the sensitive characteristic A or does not have the innocuous characteristic F, or at the same time does have neither of them.

It is clear that in any case the number reported by a person participating in such a survey is one of the numbers $0, 1, \ldots, G, G+1$. It should be emphasized that, for the method to be valid, it is crucial that the participants fully understand the meaning of the item on the list related to the stigmatizing characteristic and when this item is applicable to their case. For a person in the first sample, the item is applicable if he/she belongs to the sensitive category and or has the non-stigmatizing characteristic F. Similarly, for a person in the second sample the last item applies if he/she is not a member of the stigmatizing group or he/she does not possess the innocuous item F or if he/she does not possess the stigmatizing attribute and at the same time does not have the non-stigmatizing item F.

Let $n_k^{(1)}$ denote the number of respondents in the first sample reporting agreement with exactly k statements on the first questionnaire, with $k = 0, 1, \ldots, G+1$ and let $n_k^{(2)}$ be the corresponding number for the second sample responding to the second questionnaire. Furthermore, let p_k be the probability that exactly k of the G non-stigmatizing items are applicable to a person. Finally, let $q_k^{(1)}$ be the probability that an individual from the first sample reports agreement with k statements, and $q_k^{(2)}$ be the corresponding probability for an individual from the second sample. Then it is easy to verify that:

$$q_0^{(1)} = p_0(1-\theta)(1-\theta_F),$$
$$q_k^{(1)} = p_k(1-\theta)(1-\theta_F) + p_{k-1}(\theta + \theta_F - \theta\theta_F), \ k = 1, \ldots, G,$$
$$q_{G+1}^{(1)} = p_G(\theta + \theta_F - \theta\theta_F).$$

Similarly,

$$q_0^{(2)} = p_0\theta\theta_F,$$
$$q_k^{(2)} = p_k\theta\theta_F + p_{k-1}(1-\theta\theta_F), \ k = 1, \ldots, G,$$
$$q_{G+1}^{(2)} = p_G(1-\theta\theta_F).$$

Then $\left(n_0^{(i)}, n_1^{(i)}, \ldots, n_{G+1}^{(i)}\right)$ follows the multinomial distribution with parameters $n_i, q_0^{(i)}, \ldots, q_{G+1}^{(i)}$, for $i = 1, 2$.

6.2 The Item Count Technique

Theorem 6.1. *Let*

$$\hat{\theta} = \frac{1}{n_1}\sum_{k=0}^{G+1} k n_k^{(1)} - \frac{1}{n_2}\sum_{k=0}^{G+1} k n_k^{(2)} + 1 - \theta_F. \qquad (6.1)$$

Then $\hat{\theta}$ is unbiased for θ and its variance is given by

$$V\left(\hat{\theta}\right) = \frac{1}{n_1} Var(Z_1) + \frac{1}{n_2} Var(Z_2),$$

where Z_i is a random variable with probability mass function given by

$$P(Z_i = k) = q_k^{(i)}, \; k = 0, 1, \ldots, G+1, \; i = 1, 2.$$

Proof. Follows easily using properties of the multinomial distribution and simple algebra.

Remark 6.1. The first summation in the right-hand side of (6.1) gives the sum of the numbers reported by the respondents in the first sample while the second summation gives the corresponding number of the second sample.

Remark 6.2. Clearly, the variance of the above estimator is unknown. However, an unbiased estimator of the variance is the quantity,

$$\hat{V}\left(\hat{\theta}\right) = \frac{S_1^2}{n_1} + \frac{S_2^2}{n_2},$$

where S_1^2 and S_2^2 are the sample variances of the numbers reported by the first and second sample respectively.

The above framework is for the most convenient way to select the sample, i.e., for simple random sampling with replacement.

Assume now that using a common design p we select two independent samples s_1 and s_2 of the same average sample size, say, $v = \sum_s v(s) p(s)$, where $v(s)$ is the number of distinct units in a sample s. For a member i of the population chosen in the sample s_1, let y_i denote the number reported and let x_j denote the number reported by member j of the population chosen in the sample s_2. Let π_i (with $\pi_i > 0$) denote the inclusion probability of the person i of the population in a sample chosen according to the design p. Assume further that θ_F denotes the population proportion of people having the innocuous characteristic F which is assumed to be known. For example, θ_F may denote the population proportion of people who were born on a weekend and therefore θ_F may be taken to be $2/7$ (assuming of course that a birth takes place uniformly over all days of the week).

By applying the Horvitz–Thompson (1952) method for unbiasedly estimating a total, we may write

$$Nt_1 = t(s_1) = \sum_{i \in s_1} \frac{y_i}{\pi_i}$$

and

$$Nt_2 = t(s_2) = \sum_{j \in s_2} \frac{x_j}{\pi_j}.$$

We have the following result.

Theorem 6.2. *Let*

$$\hat{\theta} = t_1 - t_2 + 1 - \theta_F.$$

Then θ is an unbiased estimator of the population proportion θ of people having the sensitive characteristic A.

Proof. Let E_p denote the expectation operator with respect to the design p. Then

$$E_p(\hat{\theta}) = E_p(t_1) - E_p(t_2) + 1 - \theta_F$$

= {population proportion of people bearing $(A \cup F)$

in combination with $0, 1, \ldots, G$ of the G innocuous items}

−{population proportion of people bearing $(A^c \cup F^c)$

in combination with $0, 1, \ldots, G$ of the G innocuous items}

$+1 - \theta_F$

= {pop. proportion bearing A with or without any of the G items}

+{pop. proportion bearing F with or without any of the G items}

−{pop. proportion bearing A and F with or without any of the G items}

$-1 +$ {pop. proportion bearing A and F with or without any of the G items}

$+1 - \theta_F$

$= \theta + \theta_F - 1 + 1 - \theta_F$

$= \theta,$

and the proof is complete.

Let V_p denote the variance operator with respect to the design p. From Chaudhuri and Pal (2002) we know that for the total $Y = \sum_k y_k$ the variance of the Horvitz–Thompson's estimator $t(s) = \sum_{k \in s} (y_k/\pi_k)$ constructed on a sample s chosen with a design p from a population of size N is

6.2 The Item Count Technique

$$V_p(t) = \sum_{k=1}^{N} \sum_{l=k+1}^{N} (\pi_k \pi_l - \pi_{kl}) \left(\frac{y_k}{\pi_k} - \frac{y_l}{\pi_l} \right)^2 + \sum_{k=1}^{N} \frac{y_k^2}{\pi_k} \beta_k,$$

where

$$\pi_{kl} = \sum_s I_{skl} p(s), \quad \beta_k = 1 + \frac{1}{\pi_k} \sum_{l=1, l \neq k} \pi_{kl} - \nu,$$

and $I_{sij} = 1$ if both i and j belong to s and zero otherwise. An unbiased estimator of $V_p(t)$ is

$$v_p(t) = \sum_{k \in s} \sum_{l \in s, l > k} \left(\frac{\pi_k \pi_l - \pi_{kl}}{\pi_{kl}} \right) \left(\frac{y_k}{\pi_k} - \frac{y_l}{\pi_l} \right)^2 + \sum_{k \in s} \frac{y_k^2}{\pi_k^2} \beta_k,$$

assuming of course that $\pi_{ki} > 0$ for all $k \neq l$.

We immediately have the following result:

Theorem 6.3. *The variance of the estimator $\hat{\theta}$ is*

$$V_p\left(\hat{\theta}\right) = \frac{1}{N^2} \left\{ \sum_{k=1}^{N} \sum_{l=k+1}^{N} (\pi_k \pi_l - \pi_{kl}) \left[\left(\frac{y_k}{\pi_k} - \frac{y_l}{\pi_l} \right)^2 + \left(\frac{x_k}{\pi_k} - \frac{x_l}{\pi_l} \right)^2 \right] \right.$$

$$\left. + \sum_{k=1}^{N} \frac{(y_k^2 + x_k^2)}{\pi_k} \beta_k \right\}$$

and an unbiased estimator of $V_p\left(\hat{\theta}\right)$ is

$$v_p\left(\hat{\theta}\right) = \frac{1}{N^2} \left\{ \sum_{k \in s_1} \sum_{l \in s_1, l > k} \left(\frac{\pi_k \pi_l - \pi_{kl}}{\pi_{kl}} \right) \left(\frac{y_k}{\pi_k} - \frac{y_l}{\pi_l} \right)^2 \right.$$

$$+ \sum_{k \in s_2} \sum_{l \in s_2, l > k} \left(\frac{\pi_k \pi_l - \pi_{kl}}{\pi_{kl}} \right) \left(\frac{x_k}{\pi_k} - \frac{x_l}{\pi_l} \right)^2$$

$$\left. + \sum_{k \in s_1} \frac{y_k^2}{\pi_k^2} \beta_k + \sum_{k \in s_2} \frac{x_k^2}{\pi_k^2} \beta_k \right\}.$$

From the previous two theorems it is clear that the value of G in no way interferes with either the estimate or its variance. Therefore, the designer of the survey sets this value and chooses the statements about the innocuous characteristics as well as the statements which are related to the stigmatizing one. It is of course expected that the value of G is chosen wisely. The investigator should choose the value in such a way that the cooperation of the participants is secured. With this in mind, the value should not be very small or very large. In addition, the statements should be selected so that all of the values $0, 1, \ldots, G, G+1$ would be possible answers. The statement involving the stigmatizing attribute should not appear either as the first one or as the last one but it is preferable, for obvious reasons to appear somewhere in the middle. Furthermore, if the technique is incorporated into a larger questionnaire, the statements involving the G innocuous characteristics should not appear anywhere in the questionnaire and more importantly should not appear as isolated statements for which the respondent states his/her precise answer.

To increase the level of cooperation, it is suggested that the statements related to the innocuous attributes should not be totally unrelated to the stigmatizing characteristic. The respondent should have the feeling that the list serves the purpose of gathering important information on all items and that the total number reported is a meaningful number from which one can make inferences on all the items of the list.

Furthermore, it would be good to include another statement consisting of two substatements related to innocuous items, in addition to the one concerning the stigmatizing attribute.

In addition to the above, every effort should be made so that nonsampling errors are kept to a minimum. To that end, it is important that clear instructions should be given to participants so that mistakes due to misunderstanding are minimized.

Below we give such an example of sample questionnaires. These questionnaires can be utilized to estimate the prevalence of illegal doping among professional athletes in a certain community or engaging in a specific sport.

The instructions given to participants could be as follows:

"For each one of the following statements give a score of 1 in the right column if the statement applies to you and a score of 0 if not. If a statement consists of two substatements, such as Statement 2 or Statement 3, a score of 1 should be given if at least one of the substatements applies and a score of 0 if none of them does. Count the number of 1's put in the right column. This is the total score. Report the total score and nothing else. Do not return the questionnaire. It is given to you for your convenience."

	Questionnaire 1	
Number	Statement	Score
1	I am on a high protein diet.	
2	Substatement 2a: My mother was/is allergic to fish. Substatement 2b: My father was/is a smoker.	
3	Substatement 3a: I make use of illegal doping. Substatement 3b: I have taken antibiotics during last year.	
4	I have never been hospitalized.	
5	Before I became a professional athlete I used to take vitamins on a daily basis.	
6	After retirement, I will become a trainer for professional athletes.	
	Total Score:	

6.2 The Item Count Technique

\multicolumn{3}{c}{Questionnaire 2}		
Number	Statement	Score
1	I am on a high protein diet.	
2	Substatement 2a: My mother was/is allergic to fish. Substatement 2b: My father was/is a smoker.	
3	Substatement 3a: I do not make use of illegal doping. Substatement 3b: I have not taken antibiotics during last year.	
4	I have never been hospitalized.	
5	Before I became a professional athlete I used to take vitamins on a daily basis.	
6	After retirement, I will become a trainer for professional athletes.	
	Total Score:	

The previously described version of the item count technique can be applied in cases where people responding to the second questionnaire are expected to be in agreement with at least one item. Otherwise, their privacy is not protected all. A person presented with the second questionnaire who declares agreement with zero items essentially admits that he belongs to the stigmatizing category. Thus special care should be exercised when the list of statements is prepared. For the list presented above, it is expected that most people, if not all will be in agreement with at least one item. However, if there are doubts about that, then the following version should be utilized. Of course, the cost for implementing the version to be described is the need to have three independent samples.

6.2.2 Three Sample Item Count Technique

With the notation of the previous subsection, again let F denote an innocuous characteristic whose prevalence in the population is known, say θ_F. A simple random sample of size n_1 drawn with replacement from the population is given a questionnaire consisting of G innocuous items-statements and of the $(G+1)$-st item which is the following:

I have characteristic A or characteristic F.

Each respondent reports just the number of statements which are applicable to him/her, i.e., one of the numbers $0, 1, \ldots, G, G+1$ without revealing which statements are applicable to him/her. Of course, it should be explained to participants that the last statement is applicable to a person if that person has the stigmatizing characteristic A or the innocuous characteristic F or both.

A second simple random sample of size n_2 drawn with replacement from the population, independent of the first, is given a questionnaire consisting of the same G innocuous statements as the first questionnaire, and in addition a $(G+1)$-st statement which is the following:

I have characteristic A or characteristic F^c.

Again, each participant is requested to report the number of items applicable to him/her and also informed that the last item is applicable to a person if that person does have the sensitive characteristic A or characteristic F^c, or both.

Finally, a third simple random sample of size n_3 drawn with replacement from the population, independent of the first and second samples, is given a questionnaire consisting of the same G innocuous statements as the first and second questionnaires. Each participant gives the number of statements applicable to him/her.

Let $n_k^{(1)}$ and $n_k^{(2)}$ denote the number of respondents in the first and second sample, respectively, reporting agreement with exactly k statements with $k = 0, 1, \ldots, G+1$ and let $n_k^{(3)}$ be the number of people presented with the third questionnaire reporting agreement with exactly k statements with $k = 0, 1, \ldots, G$.

Again using the same notation as above, let p_k be the probability that exactly k of the G non-stigmatizing items are applicable to a person. Finally, let $q_k^{(1)}$ and $q_k^{(2)}$ be the probability that an individual from the first sample and second sample, respectively, reports agreement with k statements. Then the following are easily established:

$$q_0^{(1)} = p_0 (1-\theta)(1-\theta_F),$$
$$q_k^{(1)} = p_k (1-\theta)(1-\theta_F) + p_{k-1}(\theta + \theta_F - \theta\theta_F), \ k = 1, \ldots, G,$$
$$q_{G+1}^{(1)} = p_G (\theta + \theta_F - \theta\theta_F).$$

Similarly,

$$q_0^{(2)} = p_0 \theta_F (1-\theta),$$
$$q_k^{(2)} = p_k \theta_F (1-\theta) + p_{k-1}(\theta\theta_F + 1 - \theta_F), \ k = 1, \ldots, G,$$
$$q_{G+1}^{(2)} = p_G (\theta\theta_F + 1 - \theta_F).$$

Then $\left(n_0^{(i)}, n_1^{(i)}, \ldots, n_{G+1}^{(i)}\right)$ follows the multinomial distribution with parameters $n_i, q_0^{(i)}, \ldots, q_{G+1}^{(i)}$, for $i = 1, 2$ and $\left(n_0^{(3)}, n_1^{(3)}, \ldots, n_G^{(3)}\right)$ the multinomial distribution with parameters $n_3, p_0, \ldots, p_G$. Then using properties of the multinomial distribution one can easily prove the following result:

6.2 The Item Count Technique

Theorem 6.4. *Let*

$$\hat{\theta} = \frac{1}{n_1} \sum_{k=1}^{G+1} k n_k^{(1)} + \frac{1}{n_2} \sum_{k=1}^{G+1} k n_k^{(2)} - \frac{2}{n_3} \sum_{k=1}^{G} k n_k^{(3)} - 1.$$

Then $\hat{\theta}$ is an unbiased estimator of θ with variance

$$V\left(\hat{\theta}\right) = \frac{1}{n_1} Var(Z_1) + \frac{1}{n_2} Var(Z_2) + \frac{4}{n_3} Var(Z_3),$$

where Z_i for $i = 1, 2$ is a random variable with probability mass function given by

$$P(Z_i = k) = q_k^{(i)}, \ k = 0, 1, \ldots, G+1,$$

and Z_3 is a random variable with probability mass function given by

$$P(Z_3 = k) = p_k, \ k = 0, 1, \ldots, G.$$

Remark 6.3. Of course, the variance of the above estimator is unknown and an unbiased estimator of the variance is the quantity,

$$\hat{V}\left(\hat{\theta}\right) = \frac{S_1^2}{n_1} + \frac{S_2^2}{n_2} + \frac{4S_3^2}{n_3},$$

where S_1^2, S_2^2, and S_3^2 are the sample variances of the numbers reported by the first, second and third sample respectively.

Adopting the format of the previous subsection, the sample questionnaires can be the following:

	Questionnaire 1	
Number	Statement	Score
1	I am on a high protein diet.	
2	Substatement 2a: My mother was/is allergic to fish. Substatement 2b: My father was/is a smoker.	
3	Substatement 3a: I make use of illegal doping. Substatement 3b: I have taken antibiotics during last year.	
4	I have never been hospitalized.	
5	Before I became a professional athlete I used to take vitamins on a daily basis.	
6	After retirement, I will become a trainer for professional athletes.	
	Total Score:	

Questionnaire 2		
Number	*Statement*	*Score*
1	I am on a high protein diet.	
2	Substatement 2a: My mother was/is allergic to fish. Substatement 2b: My father was/is a smoker.	
3	Substatement 3a: I make use of illegal doping. Substatement 3b: I have not taken antibiotics during last year.	
4	I have never been hospitalized.	
5	Before I became a professional athlete I used to take vitamins on a daily basis.	
6	After retirement, I will become a trainer for professional athletes.	
	Total Score:	

Questionnaire 3		
Number	*Statement*	*Score*
1	I am on a high protein diet.	
2	Substatement 2a: My mother was/is allergic to fish. Substatement 2b: My father was/is a smoker.	
3	I have never been hospitalized.	
4	Before I became a professional athlete I used to take vitamins on a daily basis.	
5	After retirement, I will become a trainer for professional athletes.	
	Total Score:	

Remark 6.4. For the above three questionnaires clear instructions should be given to participants. See details in previous subsection.

In recent years substantial research activity has been focused on the item count technique. Pal (2007) offers a combination of randomized response with the item count technique. Hussain and Shabbir (2011) presented an item count technique approach for which only one sample is needed. Imai (2011) proposes nonlinear least squares and maximum likelihood estimators for a multivariate analysis with the item count technique.

In addition to the theoretical work on the mathematical developments of the method, various researchers and practitioners have focused on applications and various side effects. In particular Biemer and Brown (2005) observe that the method failed to produce estimates that they are higher than self-reports and they proposed a model-based estimator to correct the problem. Krebs et al. (2011) have used the technique to estimate sexual assault prevalence and to compare it with the findings of other indirect and direct estimating techniques. Tsuchiya and Hirai (2010) examine the phenomenon of underreporting which occurs according to their findings when the item count technique is applied. Finally, Coutts and Jann (2011) present experimental results for sensitive questions in online surveys to compare randomized response with the item count technique.

A further research development on the item count technique would be its implementation on estimating quantitative sensitive characteristics. Such a development would require to construct questionnaires where the nonsensitive items included represent quantitative characteristics measured on the same scale as the sensitive one. It is expected that in dealing with quantitative variables, the privacy of participants is better protected than in the case of qualitative sensitive items. In what follows, we very briefly present a version of the item count technique for quantitative stigmatizing characteristics.

6.2.3 Item Count Technique for Quantitative Sensitive Characteristics

Let μ_y be the population mean of the quantitative stigmatizing characteristic of interest. For example the stigmatizing characteristic could be the number of abortions induced, the number of times a person underreports on his/her income tax, the number of times engaged in an illegal activity, the amount of money earned and not reported etc. Our purpose is to estimate μ_y.

Assume that two independent random samples of sizes n_1 and n_2 are drawn with replacement from the population. Each one of the participants from the first sample is presented with a questionnaire (list) of $G + 1$ items, with G of those related to non-stigmatizing items and one related to the stigmatizing sensitive characteristic. All the items are quantitative in nature. The participant studies each one of the items and writes down (for his/her own convenience) the value applicable to him/her (for each one of the items). Then without reporting the individual values, he/she reports the total of all the values together. A participant from the second sample is presented with the list of the G non-stigmatizing items, exactly the same as the ones included in the questionnaire for the first sample. Again the participant is to report the total of the values applicable to him/her, without reporting the individual values. We assume that all the $G + 1$ items are independent of one another. Let $x_1, \ldots, x_G$ denote the variables representing the G nonsensitive items with $\mu_{x_1}, \ldots, \mu_{x_G}$ and $\sigma^2_{x_1}, \ldots, \sigma^2_{x_G}$ denoting the population means and variances respectively. Let also σ^2_y denote the population variance of the stigmatizing characteristic.

Let $T_1^{(1)}, \ldots, T_{n_1}^{(1)}$ and $T_1^{(2)}, \ldots, T_{n_2}^{(2)}$ be the values reported by the respondents of the first sample and second samples respectively. Let $\bar{T}^{(1)}$ and $\bar{T}^{(2)}$ denote the averages of the two samples. Then we have the following:

Theorem 6.5. *Let* $\hat{\mu}_y = \bar{T}^{(1)} - \bar{T}^{(2)}$. *Then* $\hat{\mu}_y$ *is unbiased for* μ_y *with variance*

$$V(\hat{\mu}_y) = \frac{\sigma_y^2}{n_1} + \left(\sum_{i=1}^{G} \sigma^2_{x_i}\right)\left(\frac{1}{n_1} + \frac{1}{n_2}\right). \tag{6.2}$$

Proof. It is trivial to verify that $\bar{T}^{(1)}$ unbiasedly estimates the quantity $\mu_y + \sum_{i=1}^{G} \mu_{x_i}$ and similarly that $\bar{T}^{(2)}$ is an unbiased estimator of the quantity $\sum_{i=1}^{G} \mu_{x_i}$. The variance expression follows easily given the independence of all the $G+1$ items.

The variance of the estimator is unknown. An unbiased estimator of the variance is the quantity

$$\hat{V}(\hat{\mu}_y) = \frac{S_1^2}{n_1} + \frac{S_2^2}{n_2}$$

where

$$S_k^2 = \frac{1}{n_k - 1} \sum_{i=1}^{n_k} \left(T_i^{(k)} - \bar{T}^{(k)}\right)^2, \; k = 1, 2.$$

It is important that the nonsensitive items are chosen in such a way that the possible values for those items are of the same magnitude as the possible values of the sensitive characteristic. Otherwise, the protection of privacy would be in real jeopardy.

Following are sample questionnaires for a hypothetical case where the issue is to estimate the average number of induced abortions (assuming that having an abortion is considered to be stigmatizing).

The instructions given to participants could be as follows:

"For each one of the following statements write in the right column the value applicable to you. Add all the numbers in the right column. This is your total score. Report the total score and nothing else. Do not report the individual values in the right column. Do not return the questionnaire. It is given to you for your convenience."

Questionnaire 1		
Number	Statement	Value
1	Number of uncles from my mother's side	
2	Last digit of Social Security Number	
3	Number of overseas trips taken last year	
4	Number of induced abortions	
5	Number of grandparents still alive	
	Total Score:	

Questionnaire 2		
Number	Statement	Value
1	Number of uncles from my mother's side	
2	Last digit of Social Security Number	
3	Number of overseas trips taken last year	
4	Number of grandparents still alive	
	Total Score:	

The method just presented is essentially based on masking. The participant faced with the list of the $G + 1$ statements which includes the stigmatizing one, reports the value applicable to his/her case of the variable

$$y + x_1 + \cdots + x_G.$$

But unlike other masking techniques, such as the ones by Eichhorn and Hayre (1983), Gupta, Gupta, and Singh (2002), and Huang (2010), the population means of the masking variables $x_1, \ldots, x_G$ need not be known.

The number of non-stigmatizing items should be chosen wisely. Too few or too many items will create problems. It is reasonable to assume that the more the non-stigmatizing items, the more the privacy is protected. However, as it can be seen from (6.2), inclusion of many items inflates the variance of the estimator. This is something which is not surprising, given that in indirect questioning techniques efficiency and protection of privacy move to opposite directions.

6.3 The Nominative Technique

The "Nominative Technique" introduced by Miller (1985) does not require from a respondent to disclose any sensitive information about him/her but rather to report the number of other people that the participant is close to, who possess the sensitive attribute. With the appropriate adjustment for duplicating, the investigator would be in a position to estimate the number of people in a community who belong to the stigmatizing group. The nominative methodology can be thought of as an application of network sampling introduced by Thompson (1992) and further developed by Thompson and Seber (1996) and Chaudhuri (2000). A basic prerequisite for the validity of this technique is the accurate reporting of the participants and their willingness to provide information on other members of the community that are close to them.

To develop the mathematical foundation of the method, in a population of size N, let r_{ij} for $i \neq j$ take the value 1 if the j-th participant reports that the i-th member of the population has the stigmatizing attribute and 0 otherwise. Clearly $\sum_{i=1}^{N} r_{ij}$ represents the number of people reported by the j-th participant as belonging to the stigmatizing group and similarly $\sum_{j=1}^{N} r_{ij}$ represents the number of times that the i-th member of the population is reported as having the sensitive characteristic. Finally, $\sum_{i=1}^{N} \sum_{j=1, j\neq i}^{N} r_{ij}$ gives the number of reports that persons belong to the stigmatizing group. Then the total number of people in the community having the stigmatizing attribute is given by

$$T = \sum_{i=1}^{N} \sum_{j=1, j\neq i}^{N} \left(r_{ij} / \sum_{k=1}^{N} r_{ik} \right),$$

where the quantity $r_{ij}/\sum_{k=1}^{N} r_{ik}$ is taken to be zero if $\sum_{k=1}^{N} r_{ik}$ is equal to zero. Let A_j denote the number of people belonging to the stigmatizing group reported by the j-th participant and let B_j denote the number of close friends of nominees reported by j who know that this individual belongs to the stigmatizing group. Let $x_j = A_j/(1 + B_j)$. Then

$$\hat{\theta} = \frac{1}{n}\sum_{j=1}^{n} x_j \text{ and } t = N\hat{\theta}$$

are unbiased estimators of the population proportion and population total, respectively, of the people having the sensitive attribute.

As mentioned above the nominative technique can be thought of as being an application of network sampling. We do this as follows, along the lines presented in Chaudhuri and Christofides (2008).

Assume that in a finite population of size N, we denote by N_A the number of people possessing the stigmatizing attribute. A sample of people is selected from the population and each selected person j reports about a person i in the population that he/she knows as having the sensitive characteristic. In addition, j reports the number of close friends of person i who know about the status of i as related to the stigmatizing attribute. Person i is called a "nominee" of person j. Let the participant j be referred to as a "selection unit" and "nominee" i as an "observation unit."

Let us further denote by M_j the "set" of possible nominees associated to the j-th person as close friends and let m_i be the total number of possible friends of i who are aware that this person belongs to the stigmatizing group and who might report this fact to the investigator in case they are included in the sample.

Now let the indicator $I_i(A)$ take on the value 1 if the i-th person has the sensitive attribute A and the value 0 if not. Define also,

$$y_j = \sum_{i \in M_j} \frac{I_i(A)}{m_i}$$

Then it can be easily inferred that

$$N_A = \sum_{j=1}^{N} y_i.$$

Assume that a sample s from the population is chosen with probability $p(s)$ according to a design p. Let

$$\pi_j = \sum_s I_{sj} p(s) > 0,$$

6.3 The Nominative Technique

where $I_{sj} = 1$ if $j \in s$ and zero otherwise. Let also

$$\pi_{kl} = \sum_s I_{skl} p(s) > 0,$$

where $I_{skl} = 1$ if $k, l \in s$ with $k \neq l$ and $I_{skl} = 0$ otherwise. Then

$$t = \sum_{j \in s} \frac{y_j}{\pi_j}$$

is an unbiased estimator of N_A and

$$v_p(t) = \sum_{k \in s} \sum_{l \in s, l > k} \left(\frac{\pi_k \pi_l - \pi_{kl}}{\pi_{kl}} \right) \left(\frac{y_k}{\pi_k} - \frac{y_l}{\pi_l} \right)^2 + \sum_{k \in s} \frac{y_k^2}{\pi_k^2} \beta_k$$

is an unbiased estimator of the variance of t, where

$$\beta_k = 1 + \frac{1}{\pi_k} \sum_{l=1, l \neq k}^{N} \pi_{kl} - \nu.$$

As it is expected, a person selected in the sample may "nominate" zero nominees and even all the people in the sample together may not nominate enough nominees so that the indicator function $I_i(A)$ takes on the value 1 only for a very limited number $i \in M_j$, for $j \in s$. This problem can be remedied by the adaptive sampling technique introduced by Thompson (1992) and further developed by Thompson and Seber (1996), Chaudhuri (2000), and Chaudhuri, Bose, and Ghosh (2004). The method is described briefly in what follows.

Suppose that for a selection unit j, a neighborhood is defined uniquely as the persons living in households adjacent to his/hers. If a selection unit j reports at least one nominee as having the stigmatizing characteristic, then all neighboring (to j) selection units are asked to nominate persons having the sensitive attribute. The process continues for all selection units nominating at least one person. If a selection unit gives zero nominees, then no neighboring units are asked to report any nominees. The set of selection units reached through this process initiating from the j-th one can be considered as a cluster for the j-th unit which includes itself. The selection units in the cluster that provide at least one nominee constitute a "Network" for the initial selection unit j, including j itself. All selection units left out of all such networks comprise a "singleton" network. It is clear that the entire population is the union of all the networks (including the singleton network), which of course, by construction are mutually exclusive. Let $n(j)$ denote the network of the j-th selection unit and let a_j be the cardinality of $n(j)$. Let

$$c_j = \frac{1}{a_j} \sum_{k \in n(j)} y_k.$$

Then clearly,

$$\sum_{j=1}^{N} c_j = \sum_{k=1}^{N} y_k = N_A$$

and therefore $\sum_{j \in s} (c_j/\pi_j)$ is an unbiased estimator for N_A.

The procedure described above requires that the investigator collects the information from all the selection units contained in all the networks of the selection units comprising the initial sample s. This extended sample is called the adaptive sample and the associated sampling scheme is called adaptive sampling. As one can infer, the final adaptive sample may be excessively large and the cost of implementing such a technique may be prohibitive. In order to contain the sample size so as to be cost effective, Chaudhuri, Bose, and Dihidar (2005) have developed the following procedure:

Assume that the investigator can sample up to B units of the population. Then from each $n(j)$ we take a simple random sample without replacement of size b_j such that $\sum_{j \in s} b_j \leq B$. We denote this sub-sample of $n(j)$ by $m(j)$. It is clear that this procedure requires nominations from sampling units belonging to an $m(j)$ for $j \in s$. Let

$$d_j = \frac{a_j}{b_j} \sum_{k \in m(j)} y_k.$$

Then d_j is unbiased for the quantity c_j for $j \in s$ and $\sum_{j \in s} (d_j/\pi_j)$ is unbiased for N_A. The procedure just described is termed "Restrictive Adaptive Sampling."

Remark 6.5. One may wish to estimate the number of people having the sensitive attribute and belonging to a specific subpopulation, for example we may wish to estimate the number of female persons having the sensitive characteristic. This can be easily done by utilizing appropriate indicator variables.

Although the Nominative Technique has not been used extensively, it has found its way to be applied in certain cases. Kutnik, Belser, and Danailova-Trainor (2007), although they did not use it, consider it as a good method in estimating the number of human trafficking victims. John, Edwards-Jones, Gibbons, and Jones (2010) have used it for assessing rule braking in conservation of natural resources.

6.4 The Three-Card Method

The so-called three-card method requires three independent samples. This technique, presented in Droitcour et al. (2001), is a simple technique and its name points to a technique using some devices such as boxes and cards. However, the technique, as it can be seen, can be implemented without the use of cards.

6.4 The Three-Card Method

Assume that we have three boxes, Box 1, Box 2, and Box 3. Each box contains various answer categories and the answer categories in the boxes are arranged in such a way that the sensitive item is in one of the boxes but in the company of other non-stigmatizing categories. Following Droitcour et al. (2001), let A denote the stigmatizing group, and B, C, D denote three other non-stigmatizing groups, such that the four groups are mutually exclusive. The first sample is presented with three boxes each one including statements as follows:

<u>Box 1</u>: *I belong to B.*
<u>Box 2</u>: *I belong to C or D or A.*
<u>Box 3</u>: *I belong to some other group not in Box 1 or Box 2.*

The second sample is presented with the three boxes as follows:

<u>Box 1</u>: *I belong to C.*
<u>Box 2</u>: *I belong to B or D or A.*
<u>Box 3</u>: *I belong to some other group not in Box 1 or Box 2.*

The third sample is presented with the following:

<u>Box 1</u>: *I belong to D.*
<u>Box 2</u>: *I belong to B or C or A.*
<u>Box 3</u>: *I belong to some other group not in Box 1 or Box 2.*

Each participant is instructed to report only the number of the box which is applicable to him/her. Assume that π_B, π_C, and π_D, are the population proportions of people belonging to groups B, C, D, respectively. Then it is clear that estimates $\hat{\pi}_B$, $\hat{\pi}_C$, and $\hat{\pi}_D$ of those proportions are available from the three samples. From the first sample, and using the number of people who have chosen Box 2, we can estimate the proportion of people having the stigmatizing characteristic. To that end, let $\hat{\pi}_{1CD}$ denote the proportion of the participants in the sample selecting Box 2. Then given that the groups are mutually exclusive, we immediately have that

$$\hat{\pi}_{1A} = \hat{\pi}_{1ACD} - \hat{\pi}_C - \hat{\pi}_D$$

is an estimator of the population proportion of people having the sensitive characteristic.

In the same manner, we can have two other estimators of the population proportion π_A by using the other two samples. Thus one may wish to combine the three estimators in a suitable manner. In such a case, the question arises as to how to combine the three estimators so as to have the variance of the overall estimator as small as possible. In addition, the question of optimal allocation to the three samples should be considered. It is clear that given the above considerations there is enough flexibility for the researcher to choose the appropriate sample sizes and to combine the estimators obtained from the three different samples in a wise manner.

For the three-card method to be valid, the four groups A, B, C, D must be mutually exclusive. This assumption creates an additional difficulty because the investigator must find three mutually exclusive non-stigmatizing traits, B, C, D

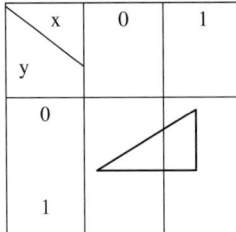 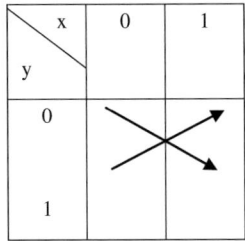

Fig. 6.1 Response structure for the triangular and cross-wise model

which in addition, are mutually exclusive with the stigmatizing trait A. This task might be proven to be difficult. In Droitcour et al. (2001) the three groups were easy to find given that the purpose was to estimate the percentage of people residing illegally in the United States (group A). Those groups were, the group of people with a valid green card issued by the U.S. government (group B), the group of people who are U.S. citizens (group C) and the group of people with a valid student or work visa (group D). However, it is really a difficult task to define the three non-stigmatizing groups in case, for example, the stigmatizing category is the group of people using illegal drugs.

6.5 Non Randomized Models

In order to guard against the pitfalls accompanying randomized response techniques, Tian, Yu, Tang, and Geng (2007), Yu, Tian, and Tang (2008) and Tan, Tian, and Tang (2009) recommended essentially the version of "Non Randomized Models" to facilitate extraction of responses on a sensitive feature say, A in the following indirect way so as to estimate the proportion bearing it in a given community of people purported to protect individual privacy to the extent possible. For an individual labeled i in the population of N people, let y_i take on the value 1 if i bears A or 0 if i bears the complement A^c; furthermore, let x_i take on the value 1 if i bears an innocuous characteristic B, say, born in one of the months August to December or the value 0 in the complimentary case B^c when i is born in one of the seven months January to July in a year.

In Fig. 6.1, the left hand side diagram gives the Triangular Structure for a possible indirect response which is either about the innocuous characteristic ($y = 0, x = 0$) or about the unrevealing one of the three alternatives ($y = 0, x = 1$), ($y = 1, x = 0$), ($y = 1, x = 1$) taken together. The two of the latter possibilities involve stigmatizing feature but not the first one. So a response "Yes"/"No" to the queries in this format need not be divulging the secret about bearing A as far as a respondent is concerned. The right hand side diagram of Fig. 6.1, on the other hand, called the "Cross-wise Model," asks a respondent either to say "Yes" about ($y = 0, x = 0$) ∪ ($y = 1, x = 1$) or about ($y = 0, x = 1$) ∪ ($y = 1, x = 0$). "Yes" response about

6.5 Non Randomized Models

either of them hides the truth about bearing A. But revelation from such responses collectively on a number of sampled persons is quite enough to provide us with the requisite estimate we need. Observe that the sample selection is only by simple random sampling with replacement for the resulting theory as propounded by Tian et al. (2007), Yu et al. (2008) and Tan et al. (2009). However, an extension to general sampling scheme is easily established as follows.

Supposing the population size N large enough, we may claim

$$\frac{1}{N}\sum_{i=1}^{N} x_i = P(x = 1) = p$$

say, and $P(x = 0) = 1 - p$, writing x for the underlying stochastic variable taking on the values $x_i, i = 1, \ldots, N$. Similarly, writing y for the sensitive variable bearing the values $y_i, i = 1, \ldots, N$, then

$$P(y = 1) = \frac{1}{N}\sum_{i=1}^{N} y_i = \theta$$

is the parameter we need to estimate. We shall assume, legitimately we may presume, that x and y are independent variables. Naturally then

$$P(y = 1, x = 1) = P(y = 1)P(x = 1) = \theta p,$$
$$P(y = 1, x = 0) = \theta(1 - p),$$
$$P(y = 0, x = 1) = (1 - \theta)p,$$
$$P(y = 0, x = 0) = (1 - \theta)(1 - p).$$

For a person labeled i, let us introduce the following notation:

$$C_{00i} = (y_i = 0, x_i = 0),$$
$$C_{01i} = (y_i = 0, x_i = 1),$$
$$C_{10i} = (y_i = 1, x_i = 0),$$
$$C_{11i} = (y_i = 1, x_i = 1).$$

Let also

$$d_i = C_{01i} \cup C_{10i} \cup C_{11i}.$$

Equivalently, we read 1 or 0 as their values if for i they hold or not. Then,

$$\frac{1}{N}\left(\sum_{i=1}^{N} C_{10i} + \sum_{i=1}^{N} C_{11i}\right) = \frac{1}{N}\sum_{i=1}^{N} y_i = \theta,$$

and

$$\frac{1}{N}\sum_{i=1}^{N} C_{00i} = (1-p)P(y=0).$$

Now,

$$\theta = \sum_{i=1}^{N} d_i - \frac{1}{N}\sum_{i=1}^{N} C_{01i}.$$

Also,

$$\frac{1}{N}\sum_{i=1}^{N} C_{01i} = \frac{p}{N}\sum_{i=1}^{N}(y_i = 0)$$

$$= pP(y=0)$$

$$= \frac{p}{1-p}\frac{1}{N}\sum_{i=1}^{N} C_{00i}.$$

From a sample s taken from the population with a probability $p(s)$ according to a general design, we have at hand the values of d_i for $i \in s$ and C_{00i} for $i \in s$. If the inclusion probabilities $\pi_i = \sum_{s \ni i} p(s)$ are all positive, then we may unbiasedly estimate θ by

$$\hat{\theta} = \frac{1}{N}\sum_{i \in s}\frac{d_i}{\pi_i} - \frac{1}{N}\frac{p}{1-p}\sum_{i \in s}\frac{C_{00i}}{\pi_i} = \frac{1}{N}\sum_{i \in s}\frac{e_i}{\pi_i},$$

where

$$e_i = d_i - \left(\frac{p}{1-p}\right)C_{00i}.$$

Supposing the general sampling design ensures each sample to have a fixed number of units, each distinct, in addition, with $\pi_{ij} = \sum_{s \ni i,j} p(s) > 0$ for every $i \neq j$, then this Horvitz–Thompson estimator $\hat{\theta}$ has the unbiased variance estimator given by Yates and Grundy (1953) as

$$u = \frac{1}{N^2}\sum_{i}\sum_{j,j>i}\left(\frac{\pi_i\pi_j - \pi_{ij}}{\pi_{ij}}\right)\left(\frac{e_i}{\pi_i} - \frac{e_j}{\pi_j}\right)^2.$$

This is for the Triangular non randomized response model. The Cross-wise model develops similarly as follows:

6.5 Non Randomized Models

For this model a response from a person i sampled in s as above will be

$$b_i = (y_i = 0, x_i = 0) \cup (y_i = 1, x_i = 1)$$

or

$$g_i = (y_i = 0, x_i = 1) \cup (y_i = 1, x_i = 0).$$

Then,

$$\frac{1}{N} \sum_{i=1}^{N} b_i = (1-p)P(y=0) + pP(y=1),$$

and

$$\frac{1}{N} \sum_{i=1}^{N} g_i = pP(y=0) + (1-p)P(y=1).$$

It follows that,

$$p\left(\frac{1}{N}\sum_{i=1}^{N} b_i\right) - (1-p)\frac{1}{N}\sum_{i=1}^{N} g_i = (2p-1)P(y=1).$$

So, $\theta = P(y=1)$ may be unbiasedly estimated by

$$\frac{1}{(2p-1)N}\left[p\sum_{i \in s}\frac{b_i}{\pi_i} - (1-p)\sum_{i \in s}\frac{g_i}{\pi_i}\right],$$

i.e., by

$$\theta^* = \frac{1}{N}\sum_{i \in s}\frac{f_i}{\pi_i}$$

where

$$f_i = \frac{pb_i - (1-p)g_i}{2p-1}$$

noting that $2p - 1 \neq 0$ since $p = 5/12$. An unbiased variance estimator for this θ^* is then

$$u^* = \frac{1}{N^2}\sum_{i \in s}\sum_{j \in s, j>i}\left(\frac{\pi_i\pi_j - \pi_{ij}}{\pi_{ij}}\right)\left(\frac{f_i}{\pi_i} - \frac{f_j}{\pi_j}\right)^2.$$

Christofides (2009) essentially provides the following indirect question and answer device avoiding any randomization experiment to be implemented by a respondent. Assume that a sample of size n is drawn with replacement from the population. Each person drawn in the sample is asked the following question:

(I) *Are you a member of (the stigmatizing) group A?*

If the answer is "Yes," without disclosing the answer, the person responds with a "Yes" or "No" to the following question:

(II) *Are you a member of (the non-stigmatizing) group B?*

Otherwise, i.e. if he/she does not have the sensitive item, he/she responds with a "Yes" or "No" to the following question:

(III) *Are you a member of (the non-stigmatizing) group C?*

The nonsensitive groups are defined by the investigator. For example B could be the group of people whose social security number ends in 5, 6, or 7 and C could be the group of people born in the months of January, February, March or April. One could also choose C to be the complement of B, as long as the population proportion of B is different from 0.5.

Assume that ϕ_1 and ϕ_2 are the known population proportions of the innocuous groups B and C, such that $\phi_1 \neq \phi_2$. It is easy to see that the probability λ of a "Yes" response from a sampled person is

$$\lambda = \theta\phi_1 + (1-\theta)\phi_2$$

from which it follows that

$$\theta = \frac{\lambda - \phi_2}{\phi_1 - \phi_2}.$$

If $\hat{\lambda}$ is the sample proportion of people providing a "Yes" response, the it is easy to show that

$$\hat{\theta} = \frac{\hat{\lambda} - \phi_2}{\phi_1 - \phi_2} \qquad (6.3)$$

is unbiased for θ with variance given by the expression

$$V\left(\hat{\theta}\right) = \frac{1}{n}\left[\frac{\theta(1-2\phi_2)}{\phi_1 - \phi_2} - \theta^2 + \frac{\phi_2(1-\phi_2)}{(\phi_1 - \phi_2)^2}\right].$$

An unbiased estimator of the variance is provided by

$$\hat{V}\left(\hat{\theta}\right) = \frac{1}{n-1}\left[\frac{\hat{\theta}(1-2\phi_2)}{\phi_1 - \phi_2} - \hat{\theta}^2 + \frac{\phi_2(1-\phi_2)}{(\phi_1 - \phi_2)^2}\right].$$

6.5 Non Randomized Models

Remark 6.6. The standard maximum likelihood estimation approach can verify that the estimator given by (6.3) is also the maximum likelihood estimator of θ. But in such a case, one ignores the possibility that the estimator produced might take on values outside the standard parameter space of the interval $[0, 1]$, and thus might exhibit the pathological symptoms of many randomized response estimators. However, by truncation we can correct the estimator so that it belongs to the correct parameter space. The truncated estimator, denoted by $\hat{\theta}_{tr}$ in this case is:

$$\hat{\theta}_{tr} = \begin{cases} 0 & \text{if } \hat{\lambda} \leq \phi_2 < \phi_1 \text{ or } \phi_1 < \phi_2 \leq \hat{\lambda} \\ \frac{\hat{\lambda} - \phi_2}{\phi_1 - \phi_2} & \text{if } \phi_2 < \hat{\lambda} < \phi_1 \text{ or } \phi_1 < \hat{\lambda} < \phi_2 \\ 1 & \text{if } \phi_2 < \phi_1 \leq \hat{\lambda} \text{ or } \hat{\lambda} \leq \phi_1 < \phi_2. \end{cases}$$

The above truncated estimator is of course biased. However, it has smaller mean squared error than the standard one.

For a general sampling design, and to keep things simple, assume that C is the complement of B and that the prevalence of B is p, with $p \neq 0.5$. Let

$$y_i = \begin{cases} 1 & \text{if } i \text{ bears } A \\ 0 & \text{if } i \text{ bears } A^c. \end{cases}$$

A sampled person is to give the response I_i which is either 1 or 0 again according to the following rule.

If i bears A, he/she is to report 1 or 0 according as he/she belongs to B; if i bears A^c he/she is to report 1 or 0 according as he/she belongs to B^c. The respondent is not to answer randomly. Yet I_i turns out to be a random variable. It has the distribution

$$P(I_i = 1) = \begin{cases} p & \text{if } i \text{ bears } A \\ 1 - p & \text{if } i \text{ bears } A^c. \end{cases}$$

So, I_i has expectation, say,

$$E_I(I_i) = y_i p + (1 - y_i)(1 - p) = (1 - p) + (2p - 1)y_i$$

and variance, say

$$V_I(I_i) = E_I(I_i)(1 - E_I(I_i)) = p(1 - p) \qquad (6.4)$$

where (6.4) follows easily since $y_i^2 = y_i$. Let

$$r_i = \frac{I_i - (1 - p)}{2p - 1}.$$

Then, $E_I(r_i) = y_i$. So, $\theta = \frac{1}{N} \sum_{i=1}^{N} y_i$ has the unbiased estimator due to Horvitz and Thompson (1952) as

$$\tilde{\theta} = \frac{1}{N} \sum_{i \in s} \frac{r_i}{\pi_i}.$$

Obviously,

$$V_i(r_i) = \frac{p(1-p)}{(2p-1)^2} = V_i,$$

say. Let us write

$$E = E_p E_I = E_I E_p$$

the overall expectation operator and

$$V = E_p V_I + V_p E_I = E_I V_p + V_I E_p$$

as the overall variance operator and taking the expectation and variance operators with respect to the sampling design as E_p and V_p, respectively. Then,

$$E\left(\tilde{\theta}\right) = \frac{1}{N} \sum_{i=1}^{N} y_i = \theta$$

giving $\tilde{\theta}$ as our required unbiased estimator for the proportion bearing A in the community of N people. Emphasizing that people report the values for I_i independently of each other implying the r_i's are independent variables, we find

$$V\left(\tilde{\theta}\right) = E_p \left(\frac{1}{N^2} \sum_{i \in s} \frac{V_i}{\pi_i^2} \right) + V_p \left(\frac{1}{N} \sum_{i \in s} \frac{y_i}{\pi_i} \right)$$

$$= \frac{1}{N^2} \left[\sum_{i \in s} \frac{V_i}{\pi_i} + \sum_{i} \sum_{j, j>i} (\pi_i \pi_j - \pi_{ij}) \left(\frac{y_i}{\pi_i} - \frac{y_j}{\pi_j} \right)^2 \right]$$

$$= E_I \left[\frac{1}{N^2} \sum_{i} \sum_{j, j>i} (\pi_i \pi_j - \pi_{ij}) \left(\frac{r_i}{\pi_i} - \frac{r_j}{\pi_j} \right)^2 + \frac{1}{N^2} \sum_{i=1}^{N} V_i \right].$$

So, an unbiased estimator for $V\left(\tilde{\theta}\right)$ is

$$v = \frac{1}{N^2} \left[\sum_{i \in s} \sum_{j \in s, j>i} \left(\frac{\pi_i \pi_j - \pi_{ij}}{\pi_{ij}} \right) \left(\frac{r_i}{\pi_i} - \frac{r_j}{\pi_j} \right)^2 + \frac{p(1-p)}{(2p-1)^2} \sum_{i \in s} \frac{1}{\pi_i} \right].$$

6.5 Non Randomized Models

Christofides' (2009) non randomized response model theoretically is quite analogous to Warner's (1965) randomized response model. The difference is on the way the randomization is performed. In Warner's (1965) technique the randomization takes place with the use of a randomization device. In Christofides' (2009) model the sensitive question is used to perform a randomization without the need of a device.

Christofides' (2009) non randomized response model is very different from the three other non randomized response models. But all four non-randomized response models discussed require the knowledge of p. However, the following modification in the previously described technique handles the case where one needs to use in the sample survey the innocuous characteristic B whose prevalence p is unknown. To keep things simple we will present the modification for the case of simple random sampling with replacement.

Again, assume that θ is the population proportion of people belonging to the sensitive group, p is the (unknown) population prevalence of the innocuous characteristic B and ϕ be the known prevalence of the innocuous characteristic C, assuming that $\phi \neq 0.5$. We need to draw two independent random samples of sizes n_1 and n_2. Each person from the first sample is faced with the following question:

(I) *Are you a member of (the stigmatizing) group A?*

If the answer is "Yes," without disclosing his/her answer to the interviewer, the sampled person responds with a "Yes" or "No" to the following question:

(II) *Are you a member of (the non-stigmatizing) group B?*

Otherwise, i.e. if he/she does not belong to group A, he/she is to provide a "Yes" or "No" answer to the question:

(III) *Are you a member of (the non-stigmatizing) group C?*

For people drawn in the second sample the procedure is the same except that question (III) is replaced by the following question:

(IV) *Are you a member of (the non-stigmatizing) group C^c?*

Let λ_1 and λ_2 be the probability of a "Yes" response from a person sampled in the first and second sample respectively. Then

$$\lambda_1 = \theta p + (1-\theta)\phi \text{ and } \lambda_2 = \theta p + (1-\theta)(1-\phi). \tag{6.5}$$

From these two equations we immediately have that

$$\theta = 1 - \frac{\lambda_1 - \lambda_2}{2\phi - 1}.$$

Based on that and assuming that $\hat{\lambda}_1$ and $\hat{\lambda}_2$ are the sample proportions of people providing a "Yes" response, we can show that is an unbiased estimator of θ with variance

$$V\left(\hat{\theta}\right) = \frac{1}{(2\phi-1)^2}\left[\frac{\lambda_1(1-\lambda_1)}{n_1} + \frac{\lambda_2(1-\lambda_2)}{n_2}\right].$$

An unbiased estimator of the variance is provided by

$$\hat{V}\left(\hat{\theta}\right) = \frac{1}{(2\phi-1)^2}\left[\frac{\hat{\lambda}_1\left(1-\hat{\lambda}_1\right)}{n_1-1} + \frac{\hat{\lambda}_2\left(1-\hat{\lambda}_2\right)}{n_2-1}\right].$$

$$\hat{\theta} = 1 - \frac{\hat{\lambda}_1 - \hat{\lambda}_2}{2\phi - 1}$$

Observe that based on this method, one can also estimate the prevalence p of the nonsensitive characteristic B by means of any one of Eq. (6.5).

The previously modified version of the device free randomized response model could be applied for estimating the percentage of students engaging in a specific form of academic dishonesty. What follows is a "hypothetical" example where we focus on estimating the percentage of senior undergraduate students (of a specific university) who have applied, at least once during the course of their studies for outside (paid) help in order to prepare an essay or a project needed as part of their homework assignment. Obviously, the issue is sensitive enough and therefore, direct responses are difficult to obtain, and even in case one is able to collect answers, they are likely to be untruthful. Assume that two random samples of sizes 154 and 138 of senior undergraduate students were selected. The students are instructed to submit their answer on a specifically designed web page, which is accessible only to them. In the instructions, it is explained what the purpose of the survey is and that the method does not allow for anyone to infer whether each one of them personally has engaged in the specific activity of plagiarism. The specific instructions (related to the method) for each student selected in the first sample are the following:

> "If during the course of your studies you have paid at least once an outsider to prepare for you a homework assignment, answer the following question A with a "Yes" or "No." Otherwise, answer question B.
>
> > Question A: *If you were to begin your studies again, would you choose this University for your undergraduate studies?*
> > Question B: *Is the last digit of the last outgoing call from your mobile phone, 6, or 7 or 8 or 9?*

The instructions for each student selected in the second sample were the following:

> "If during the course of your studies you have paid at least once an outsider to prepare for you a homework assignment, answer the following question A with a "Yes" or "No." Otherwise, answer question B.

6.5 Non Randomized Models

Question A: *If you were to begin your studies again, would you choose this University for your undergraduate studies?*
Question B: *Is the last digit of the last outgoing call from your mobile phone, 0, or 1, or 2, or 3, or 4, or 5?*

Suppose that at the end of this survey, 39 of the students in the first sample gave a "Yes" response (and 115 a "No" response) while for the second sample 43 "Yes" and 95 "No" responses are recorded. In this scenario, group C is the group of people whose last outgoing call ends in 6, 7, 8, or 9. Assuming that outgoing calls from someone's mobile phone are equally likely to end in any of the ten digits, then $\phi = 0.4$. From the previous data, we find that

$$\hat{\lambda}_1 = \frac{39}{154} \approx 0.25 \text{ and } \hat{\lambda}_2 = \frac{43}{138} \approx 0.31.$$

Then the point estimate of θ is

$$\hat{\theta} = 1 - \frac{\hat{\lambda}_1 - \hat{\lambda}_2}{2\phi - 1} = 1 - \frac{0.25 - 0.31}{0.8 - 1} = 0.7$$

with estimated variance

$$\hat{V}\left(\hat{\theta}\right) = \frac{1}{(2\phi - 1)^2} \left[\frac{\hat{\lambda}_1 \left(1 - \hat{\lambda}_1\right)}{n_1 - 1} + \frac{\hat{\lambda}_2 \left(1 - \hat{\lambda}_2\right)}{n_2 - 1} \right]$$

$$= \frac{1}{(0.2)^2} \left[\frac{0.25(1 - 0.25)}{153} + \frac{0.31(1 - 0.31)}{137} \right]$$

$$\approx 0.07,$$

i.e., the point estimate for the percentage of senior students engaging in this sensitive activity is estimated to be around 70 %, with estimated variance 7 %. From the data it is also possible to estimate the percentage of senior students who would choose another institution for their studies, if they were to start from the very beginning. This percentage is found to be around 80 %. These figures, although are based on hypothetical data and even in case of real data the estimates are subject to various forms of nonsampling error, it is possible that are not far from reality. There are many studies, some of them utilizing indirect questioning techniques which prove that plagiarism and academic dishonesty in universities is widespread. See for example, Coutts, Jann, Krumpal, and Naeher (2011), Jann, Jerke, and Krumpal (2012) and Hejri, Zendehdel, Asghari, Fotouhi, and Rashidian (2013).

Further details on the non randomized models presented in this section can be found in Chaudhuri (2012).

6.6 Surveys with Negative Questions

Surveys with negative questions or simply "negative surveys" have been introduced initially by Esponda (2006) and later developed by Esponda and Guerrero (2009). The technique is relatively new and further research on this area is expected to follow in the years to come. The technique combines elements of direct survey research and randomized response. Following Esponda and Guerrero (2009) consider the following scenario.

Assume that we have a survey questionnaire which consists of a single question. To this question a participant provides one answer from a list of k possible answers. These answers must be mutually exclusive and exhaustive, i.e., the participant must provide only one answer and precisely one applies to him/her. This scenario is the typical scenario of direct questionnaires, although it is not realistic to assume that the entire questionnaire consists of a single question. In case the question is of sensitive nature, the survey exhibits the usual pathology of direct questioning. Let us call a survey utilizing such a questionnaire a "positive question survey." For example, following Esponda and Guerrero (2009), assume that the questionnaire consists of the following item:

I earn:

(a) *Less than 30000 euros a year*
(b) *Between 30000 and 70000 euros a year*
(c) *More than 70000 euros a year.*

The purpose of such a questionnaire is to estimate, based on a simple random sample of size n chosen with replacement from the population the proportion of people belonging to each one of the three income categories.

Now consider a questionnaire, the negative of the above, which again consists of a single question with k possible answers, all of which, except one (and only one) are true for each participant. The participant is requested to report to the interviewer one of the true ones. The question is phrased in a negative manner and by reporting a specific answer, the participant provides a category to which he/she does not belong. For the above questionnaire, its negative is the following:

I do not earn:

(a) *Less than 30000 euros a year*
(b) *Between 30000 and 70000 euros a year*
(c) *More than 70000 euros a year.*

It is clear that for a participant, two out of the three options are valid. For example, a person whose income is more than 70,000 euros should report either (a) or (b).

For the above approach, Esponda and Guerrero (2009) argue that by utilizing Shannon's uncertainty measure, one can show what the intuition points out to, namely that the amount of information disclosed by answering a questionnaire containing the "negative question" is no more than the amount of information

6.6 Surveys with Negative Questions

disclosed when responding to the direct version of the questionnaire. To that end, let X be the random variable representing the true category of a member of the population. Let also $\pi_i = P(X = i)$ be the probability that category i is true in a direct response survey and let $P(X = i | X \neq s)$ be the probability that category i is true after s has been removed, i.e., after finding out that it is not applicable. Then the information disclosed by answering the negative questionnaire can be expressed as

$$I(1,\ldots,k|X \neq s) = -\sum_{i=1}^{k}\pi_i \log \pi_i + \sum_{i \neq s} P(X = i|X \neq s) \log P(X = i|X \neq s).$$

The first term of the right-hand side is the amount of information disclosed from the positive version of the questionnaire and the second term is the amount of information from the same questionnaire, after category s is no longer an option. From the above equation it is clear that

$$I(1,\ldots,k|X \neq s) \leq -\sum_{i=1}^{k}\pi_i \log \pi_i,$$

showing that the amount of information disclosed from the negative questionnaire, is at most the amount of information disclosed by responding to the positive one.

As above, let X be the random variable representing the true category of a member of the population. In addition let Y be the random variable representing the reported category. Assume further that

$$P(Y = i) = \lambda_i, \; i = 1, \ldots, k$$

and that the quantities $\lambda_1, \ldots, \lambda_k$ are the same for all participants. Let also n_i denote the number of times the event $\{Y = i\}$ occurs. Then the random vector $(n_1, \ldots, n_k)^T$ follows the multinomial distribution with parameters n and $\underline{\lambda} = (\lambda_1, \ldots, \lambda_k)^T$. Let

$$p_{ii} = 0,$$
$$p_{ij} = P(Y = i | X = j), \text{ for } i \neq j.$$

Then we can express the probability λ_i as

$$\lambda_i = \sum_{j=1}^{k} P(Y=i|X=j)\pi_j = \sum_{j=1}^{k} p_{ij}\pi_j, \; i = 1, \ldots, k. \tag{6.6}$$

Equation (6.6) can be written in matrix notation as

$$\underline{\lambda} = \mathbf{P}\underline{\pi},$$

where **P** is a k-dimensional square matrix with elements the quantities p_{ij} and $\underline{\pi} = (\pi_1, \ldots, \pi_k)^T$.

It is known that the maximum likelihood estimator of the probability λ_i is the sample proportion $\hat{\lambda}_1 = n_i/n$ and by utilizing properties of the multinomial distribution we immediately have that

$$E\left(\hat{\lambda}_i\right) = \lambda_i,$$

$$\text{Var}\left(\hat{\lambda}_i\right) = \frac{\lambda_i(1-\lambda_i)}{n}, \; i = 1, \ldots, k$$

and

$$\text{Cov}\left(\hat{\lambda}_i, \hat{\lambda}_j\right) = -\frac{\lambda_i \lambda_j}{n}, i = 1, \ldots, k, \; j = 1, \ldots, k, \; i \neq j.$$

The following theorem of Esponda and Guerrero (2009) whose proof is similar to the one with **P** not necessarily a square matrix, presented in Chaudhuri and Mukerjee (1988), p. 37, gives an unbiased estimator for the vector $\underline{\pi} = (\pi_1, \ldots, \pi_k)^T$.

Theorem 6.6. *If the matrix* **P** *is nonsingular, an unbiased estimator of $\underline{\pi}$ is the quantity $\hat{\underline{\pi}} = \mathbf{P}^{-1}\hat{\underline{\lambda}}$ with variance*

$$\text{Var}\left(\hat{\underline{\pi}}\right) = \frac{1}{n}\mathbf{P}^{-1}\left[\text{Diag}(\underline{\lambda}) - \underline{\lambda}\underline{\lambda}^T\right]\left(\mathbf{P}^T\right)^{-1}$$

where $\hat{\underline{\lambda}} = \left(\hat{\lambda}_1, \ldots, \hat{\lambda}_k\right)^T$ and Diag $(\underline{\lambda})$ is a diagonal matrix with $\lambda_1, \ldots, \lambda_k$ as its diagonal elements.

It is reasonable to expect that in a questionnaire with negative questions, a respondent is biased against options which might be considered as stigmatizing. For the above scenario with the income example, a person earning between 30,000 and 70,000 euros is more likely to choose option (c) than option (a). Therefore the issue of how participants choose an option is of major significance. One possibility is that participants are instructed to choose any option with the same probability, for example with the use of a fair die having $k-1$ faces. Another possibility would be to give instructions to the participants to select an option with different probabilities with the use of a die manufactured for that purpose. Xie, Kulik, and Tanin (2011) propose the use of the so-called Gaussian Negative Surveys, where the selection of the response is based on the normal distribution. In any case, this is an issue that needs to be further studied and developed.

For the case where each one of the other $k-1$ options is selected with the same probability, i.e., when

$$p_{ii} = 0,$$

$$p_{ij} = P(Y = i | X = j) = \frac{1}{k-1} \text{ for } i \neq j,$$

following Esponda and Guerrero (2009) we say that we have the equal chance design. For that design we have the following result, due to Esponda and Guerrero (2009).

Theorem 6.7. *Assume that we have the equal chance design. Then an unbiased estimator for the population proportion π_i is given by*

$$\hat{\pi}_i = 1 - (k-1)\hat{\lambda}_i$$

where $\hat{\lambda}_i = n_i/n$ for $i = 1, \ldots, k$ with variance

$$Var(\hat{\pi}_i) = \frac{\pi_i(1-\pi_i)}{n}\left(1 + \frac{k-2}{\pi_i}\right).$$

Observe that in the above formula for the variance of the estimator, the first factor is the variance that one would have if a direct survey is conducted, and the second part is the price we pay for using the randomization. From the above expression for the variance it is clear that the number of options should be kept to a minimum, i.e., it should be as small as possible. Of course, it is obvious that in case $k = 2$ the second part does not exist, but after all, in such a case, we do not have a survey with negative questions but we essentially have a direct survey with only two options for the original question.

Variations of surveys with negative questions can be described and studied. Some of them follow directly from the material in Esponda (2006) and Esponda and Guerrero (2009). Some others can be further developed, for example the case where a participant has the option to use the questionnaire with the direct question or the questionnaire with the negative version. In such a case, based on the experience from the similar approach in randomized response, one expects to obtain estimates with lower mean square error. Obviously, it will be difficult if not impossible to use surveys with negative questions in order to estimate purely qualitative characteristics.

References

Biemer, P., & Brown, G. (2005). Model-based estimation of drug prevalence using item count data. *Journal of Official Statistics, 21,* 287–308.

Chaudhuri, A. (2000). Network and adaptive sampling with unequal probabilities. *Calcutta Statistical Association Bulletin, 50,* 237–253.

Chaudhuri, A. (2012). Unbiased estimation of a sensitive proportion in general sampling by three non-randomized response schemes. *Journal of Statistical Theory and Practice, 6,* 376–381.

Chaudhuri, A., Bose, M., Dihidar, K. (2005). Sample size restrictive adaptive sampling: an application in estimating localized elements. *Journal of Statistical Planning and Inference, 134,* 254–267.

Chaudhuri, A., Bose, M., Ghosh, J.K. (2004). An application of adaptive sampling to estimate highly localized population segments. *Journal of Statistical Planning and Inference, 121*, 175–189.

Chaudhuri, A., & Christofides, T.C. (2007). Item count technique in estimating the proportion of people with a sensitive feature. *Journal of Statistical Planning and Inference, 137*, 589–593.

Chaudhuri, A., & Christofides, T.C. (2008). Indirect questioning: how to rival randomized response techniques. *International Journal of Pure and Applied Mathematics, 43*, 283–294.

Chaudhuri, A., & Mukerjee, R. (1988). *Randomized response: theory and techniques*. New York: Marcel Dekker.

Chaudhuri, A., & Pal, S. (2002). On certain alternative mean square error estimators in complex survey sampling. *Journal of Statistical Planning and Inference, 104*, 363–375.

Christofides, T.C. (2009). Randomized response without a randomization device. *Advances and Applications in Statistics, 11*, 15–28.

Coutts, E., & Jann, B. (2011). Sensitive questions in online surveys: experimental results for the randomized response technique (RRT) and the unmatched count technique (UCT). *Sociological Methods & Research, 40*, 169–193.

Coutts, E., Jann, B., Ivar, K., Anatol-Fiete, N. (2011). Plagiarism in student papers: prevalence estimates using special techniques for sensitive questions. *Journal of Economics and Statistics, 231*, 749–760.

Droitcour, J.A., Larson, E.M., Scheuren, F.J. (2001). The three card method: estimating sensitive items with permanent anonymity of response. In *Proceedings of the Social Statistics Section of the American Statistical Association*. Alexandria, VA: ASA.

Eichhorn, B.H., & Hayre, L.S. (1983). Scrambled randomized response methods for obtaining quantitative data. *Journal of Statistical Planning and Inference, 7*, 306–316.

Esponda, F. (2006). Negative surveys. arXiv:ST/0608176v1

Esponda, F., & Guerrero, V.M. (2009). Surveys with negative questions for sensitive items. *Statistics and Probability Letters, 79*, 2456–2461.

Gupta, S., Gupta, B., Singh, S. (2002). Estimation of sensitivity level of personal interview survey question. *Journal of Statistical Planning and Inference, 100*, 239–247.

Hejri, M.S., Zendehdel, K., Asghari, F., Fotouhi, A., Rashidian, A. (2013). Academic disintegrity among medical students: a randomized response technique study. *Medical Education, 47*, 144–153.

Horvitz, D.G., & Thompson, D.J. (1952). A generalization of sampling without replacement from finite universe. *Journal of the American Statistical Association, 47*, 663–685.

Huang, K.-C. (2010). Unbiased estimators of mean, variance and sensitivity level for quantitative characteristics in finite population sampling. *Metrika, 71*, 341–352.

Hussain, Z., & Shabbir, J. (2011). On item count technique in survey sampling. *Journal of Informatics and Mathematical Sciences, 2*, 161–169.

Imai, K. (2011). Multivariate regression analysis for the item count technique. *Journal of the American Statistical Association, 106*, 407–415.

Jann, B., Jerke, J., Krumpal, I. (2012). Asking sensitive questions using the crosswise model: an experimental survey measuring plagiarism. *Public Opinion Quarterly, 76*, 32–49.

John, F.A.V. St., Edwards-Jones, G., Gibbons, J.M., Jones, J.P.G. (2010). Testing novel methods for assessing rule breaking in conservation. *Biological Conservation, 143*, 1025–1030.

Krebs, C.P., Lindquist, C.H., Warner, T.D., Fisher, B.S., Martin, S.L., Childers, J.M. (2011). Comparing sexual assault prevalence estimates obtained with direct and indirect questioning techniques. *Violence Against Women, 17*, 219–235.

Kutnik, B., Belser, P., Danailova-Trainor, G. (2007). Methodologies for global and national estimation of human trafficking victims: current and future approaches. In *Working paper 29*, International Labour Office, Geneva.

Miller, J.D. (1984). *A new survey technique for studying deviant behavior*. Ph.D. Thesis, The George Washington University.

Miller, J.D. (1985). The nominative technique: a new method of estimating heroin prevalence. *NIDA Research Monograph*, No. 57, 104–124.

Miller, J.D., Cisin, I.H., Harrel, A.V. (1986). A new technique for surveying deviant behavior: item count estimates of marijuana, cocaine and heroin. *Paper presented at the annual meeting of the American Association for Public Opinion Research*, St. Petersburg, Florida.

Pal, S. (2007). Estimating the proportion of people bearing a sensitive issue with an option to item count lists and randomized response. *Statistics in Transition*, *8*, 301–310.

Raghavarao, D., & Federer, W.F. (1979). Block total response as an alternative to the randomized response method in surveys. *Journal of the Royal Statistical Society: Series B*, *41*, 40–45.

Tan, M.T., Tian, G.L., Tang, M.L. (2009). Sample surveys with sensitive questions: a non-randomized response approach. *American Statistician*, *63*, 9–16.

Tian, G.-L., Yu, J.-W., Tang, M.-L., Geng, Z. (2007). A new nonrandomized model for analyzing sensitive questions with binary outcomes. *Statistics in Medicine*, *26*, 4238–4252.

Thompson, S.K. (1992). *Sampling*. New York: Wiley.

Thompson, S.K., & Seber, G.A.F. (1996). *Adaptive sampling*. New York: Wiley.

Tsuchiya, T., & Hirai, Y. (2010). Elaborate item count questioning: why do people underreport in item count responses? *Survey Research Methods*, *4*, 139–149.

Yates, F., & Grundy, P.M. (1953). Selection without replacement from within strata with probability proportional to size. *Journal of the Royal Statistical Society: Series B*, *15*, 253–261.

Yu, J.-W., Tian, G.-L., Tang, M.-L. (2008). Two new models for survey sampling with sensitive characteristic: design and analysis. *Metrika*, *67*, 251–263.

Warner, S.L. (1965). Randomized response: a survey technique for eliminating evasive answer bias. *Journal of the American Statistical Association*, *60*, 63–69.

Xie, H., Kulik, L., Tanin, E. (2011). Privacy-aware collection of aggregate spatial data. *Journal of Data and Knowledge Engineering*, *70*, 576–595.

Chapter 7
Protection of Privacy

Abstract The main motivation behind indirect questioning is to increase participation, reduce nonresponse and reduce untruthful responses in surveys dealing with stigmatizing characteristics. Indirect questioning techniques are often advertised as methods protecting the privacy of the participants in surveys dealing with stigmatizing or sensitive issues. This is easy for anyone to see. However, different techniques do not necessarily offer the same level of protection. Quantitative measures of the protection of privacy and measures of jeopardy have been devised, which can be used, among other things, to compare one indirect questioning technique to another. Those measures are discussed and special emphasis is put on their limitations. In this chapter a case is made for the need to develop quantitative measures of the protection of privacy as perceived by the participants. A person is willing to participate in indirect questioning sample surveys if he/she feels that his/her privacy is protected and that the answer provided is not sufficient for someone to determine whether he/she bears the stigmatizing characteristic. Real life examples are cited which prove that the issue of privacy protection from the participant's point of view is indeed very important.

7.1 Introduction

Responding to questions of sensitive nature may jeopardize one's privacy. In fact the need to develop the randomized response methodology was founded on the purpose to protect the privacy and anonymity of the participants so that the percentage of people refusing to respond or providing untruthful responses is appreciably limited to a minimum. Various mathematical measures of protection of privacy have been developed. Those measures can be assessed in relation to the efficiency for each one of the randomized response techniques. In general, the privacy protection measures and the efficiency of a technique move to opposite directions.

In addition, the measures of the protection of privacy are mathematical objects which cannot be easily (if not at all) understood by the participants. Respondents' criterion for participation in an indirect questioning survey is what one may call the perceived protection of privacy, i.e., their own subjective measure of how their anonymity is maintained and their own feeling of how their privacy is protected.

In Sect. 7.2 we present the measures of jeopardy for indirect questioning and in particular for randomized response techniques. The issue of efficiency and protection of privacy is examined. In Sect. 7.3 we discuss the issue of privacy protection in randomized response techniques for quantitative stigmatizing characteristics. In Sect. 7.4 we examine the issue of the perception of privacy protection and provide evidence that the perceived protection of privacy and privacy protection do not always coincide. Finally, we make a case for further development and study of the issue of the perceived protection of privacy.

7.2 Measures of Jeopardy

Measures of the protection of privacy associated with randomized response techniques have been devised and presented by various authors. For a brief summary of those measures one may consult Ljungqvist (1993), although new measures and approaches have been presented more recently. See, for example, Guerriero and Sandri (2007), Quatember (2009), Nayak and Adeshiyan (2009), Chaudhuri, Christofides, and Saha (2009) and Hong, Yan, and Wei (2010). It has to be noted, however, that no measure of privacy protection is universally accepted. For each one of the measures of privacy protection one can point out its limitations and disadvantages.

Assume that θ denotes the probability that a person belongs to a sensitive or stigmatizing group A. Let R denote a specific response by a person participating in a randomized response survey. The quantity $P(A|R)$ denotes the probability that a person has the stigmatizing characteristic given that his/her response is R and similarly $P(A^c|R)$ denotes the probability that he/she does not belong to the stigmatizing group given that the response provided is R. Then

$$P(A|R) = \frac{\theta P(R|A)}{\theta P(R|A) + (1-\theta) P(R|A^c)} \tag{7.1}$$

and

$$P(A^c|R) = \frac{(1-\theta) P(R|A^c)}{\theta P(R|A) + (1-\theta) P(R|A^c)} \tag{7.2}$$

are considered as revealing probabilities as to whether a person belongs to A or to A^c when he/she provides the specific response R. One may say that the privacy is protected if the conditional probability of a person belonging to the stigmatizing group given that the response provided is R is no greater than the prior probability θ. Based on this approach we may consider the response R as jeopardizing with respect

7.2 Measures of Jeopardy

to A if $P(A|R) > \theta$. Similarly, R is jeopardizing with respect to A^c if $P(A^c|R) > 1 - \theta$. If we combine (7.1) and (7.2), then

$$J(R) = \frac{P(A|R)/\theta}{P(A^c|R)/(1-\theta)} = \frac{P(R|A)}{P(R|A^c)}$$

can be thought of as a measure of jeopardy and high values of this measure indicate that the protection of privacy of a respondent is in jeopardy. The above measure is due to Leysieffer and Warner (1976).

The conditional probabilities in (7.1) and (7.2) can be used to compare two different randomized response techniques, say Technique 1 and Technique 2. Following Lanke (1976) we can define the quantity

$$g(A) = \max\{P(A|R=1), P(A|R=0)\}.$$

Then we say that Technique 1 is more protective than Technique 2 if $g(A)$ for Technique 1 is smaller than $g(A)$ for Technique 2. For such a comparison of course, one should also account for the efficiency between the two techniques.

Nayak (1994) studied extensively the measures of privacy protection. His approach is to use the probabilities $P(A|R=1)$ and $P(A|R=0)$ in order to compare two different randomized response techniques. To that end, he states that design d_1 is better than design d_2 if

$$P_{d_1}(A|R=1) \leq P_{d_2}(A|R=1),$$
$$P_{d_1}(A|R=0) \leq P_{d_2}(A|R=0),$$

and

$$V_{d_1}\left(\hat{\theta}\right) \leq V_{d_2}\left(\hat{\theta}\right),$$

for all $\theta \in [0, 1]$ and at least one strict inequality holds for some θ, where the subscripts d_1 and d_2 specify the design. However Nayak's presentation as well as of his predecessors is focused on the case where the respondents are selected using simple random sampling with replacement. Chaudhuri and Saha (2004) and Chaudhuri et al. (2009) covered the situation where respondents are selected with a general sampling scheme. We will describe this latter approach later on in this chapter. First, we will present an interesting method to compare the efficiency of methods offering the same protection of privacy. This method is due to Quatember (2009).

Quatember's approach is first to describe a number of randomized response techniques in a unified manner, termed by him as standardization. Assume again that A denotes the stigmatizing group, whereas B denotes an innocuous group, such as the one used in Greenberg et al.'s (1969) Unrelated Question Model.

Each respondent is instructed to do one of the following five things, with respective probabilities p_1, p_2, p_3, p_4, p_5, such that $\sum_{i=1}^{5} p_i = 1$.

(a) To answer with "Yes" or "No" the question: *Are you a member of group A?*
(b) To answer with "Yes" or "No" the question: *Are you a member of group A^c?*
(c) To answer with "Yes" or "No" the question: *Are you a member of group B?*
(d) To say "Yes."
(e) To say "No."

By assigning to some of the parameters p_1, p_2, p_3, p_4, p_5, the values zero and one we can have specific techniques known in the literature. For example if $p_1 = 1$ then what we have is just a direct questioning survey. By choosing $p_3 = p_4 = p_5 = 0$ we have the standard Warner's (1965) technique, while by choosing $p_2 = p_4 = p_5 = 0$ we have Greenberg et al.'s (1969) Unrelated Question Model. This standardization contains 16 different models. Let as before θ denote the population proportion of people belonging to the sensitive group A and θ_B denote the population proportion of people having the nonsensitive characteristic B. Let the variable y_i take on the value 1 if the i-th unit of the population U has the sensitive characteristic and the value 0 otherwise. Let also the variable z_i be equal to 1 if the i-th unit of the sample answers "Yes" and the value 0 otherwise. Then the probability of a "Yes" answer with respect to the randomized response questioning design R is:

$$P_R(z_i = 1) = p_1 y_i + p_2(1 - y_i) + p_3 \theta_B + p_4 = a y_i + b$$

where $a = p_1 - p_2$ and $b = p_2 + p_3 \theta_B + p_4$. Then it is trivial to verify that $\hat{y}_i = a^{-1}(z_i - b)$ unbiasedly estimates y_i provided $a \neq 0$, and consequently, for a sampling design with inclusion probabilities π_i, the quantity

$$\hat{\theta} = \frac{1}{N} \sum_s \frac{\hat{y}_i}{\pi_i} \tag{7.3}$$

unbiasedly estimates θ where N is the size of the population. For a probability sampling design p, the variance of the estimator is given by

$$V_p(\hat{\theta}) = \frac{1}{N^2} \left[V_p \left(\sum_{i \in s} \frac{y_i}{\pi_i} \right) + \frac{b(1-b)}{a^2} \sum_{i \in U} \frac{1}{\pi_i} + \frac{1 - 2b - a}{a} \sum_{i \in U} \frac{y_i}{\pi_i} \right]. \tag{7.4}$$

This variance is of course unknown and unbiased estimators can be obtained by replacing $V_p \left(\sum_s (y_i/\pi_i) \right)$ by an unbiased estimator $\hat{V}_p \left(\sum_s (y_i/\pi_i) \right)$ and the term $\sum_U (y_i/\pi_i)$ by $\sum_U (\hat{y}_i/\pi_i^2)$. In the special case where the sampling design is simple random sampling without replacement, (7.3) and (7.4) are respectively

$$\hat{\theta} = \frac{\hat{\pi}_{yes} - b}{a}$$

7.2 Measures of Jeopardy

and

$$V\left(\hat{\theta}\right) = \frac{N-n}{N-1}\frac{\theta(1-\theta)}{n} + \frac{1}{n}\left(\frac{b(1-b)}{a^2} + \frac{(1-2b-a)\theta}{a}\right),$$

where $\hat{\pi}_{yes}$ is the proportion of people responding "Yes" in the sample of size n. This variance of course can be unbiasedly estimated by

$$\hat{V}\left(\hat{\theta}\right) = \frac{\hat{\theta}\left(1-\hat{\theta}\right)(N-n)}{(n-1)N} + \frac{1}{n}\left(\frac{b(1-b)}{a^2} + \frac{(1-2b-a)\hat{\theta}}{a}\right).$$

The above expression of the variance can be used to compare the efficiency of the various randomized response techniques which can be described by the general standardized model, provided they offer the same level of privacy protection. Again following Quatember (2009), consider the following measures of privacy.

$$\lambda_j = \frac{\max\{P(z_i = j \mid i \in A),\ P(z_i = j \mid i \in A^c)\}}{\min\{P(z_i = j \mid i \in A),\ P(z_i = j \mid i \in A^c)\}},\ j = 0, 1.$$

Expressing the parameters λ_0 and λ_1 in terms of the quantities a and b we have the alternative expressions

$$\lambda_0 = \frac{\max\{1-a-b,\ 1-b\}}{\min\{1-a-b,\ 1-b\}} \tag{7.5}$$

and

$$\lambda_1 = \frac{\max\{a+b,\ b\}}{\min\{a+b,\ b\}}. \tag{7.6}$$

The quantities λ_0 and λ_1 can take on any value from 1 to infinity. The privacy is completely protected in the extreme case where the two parameters are equal to 1. But in such a case, the answer of the participants is not informative and thus useless. Higher values of these two measures imply more information on the sensitive characteristic, but as is always the case, this results in loss of efficiency.

From (7.5) and (7.6) one can express the quantities a and b in terms of the measures λ_0 and λ_1. By doing so, one has

$$a = \frac{\left(1-\lambda_1^{-1}\right)\left(1-\lambda_0^{-1}\right)}{1-\lambda_0^{-1}\lambda_1^{-1}} \quad \text{and} \quad b = \frac{\lambda_1^{-1}\left(1-\lambda_0^{-1}\right)}{1-\lambda_0^{-1}\lambda_1^{-1}}.$$

Then, it follows that the variance of the estimator for a sampling design p depends on the loss of privacy which is measured by the quantities λ_0 and λ_1. Thus, designs with the same values for λ_0 and λ_1 are equally efficient. Given that, one could choose the design parameters in an optimal way so as to achieve the prescribed levels of λ_0 and λ_1. For example, for Warner's (1965) technique, choosing $p_1 = \lambda_1/(1 + \lambda_1)$ and $p_2 = 1 - p_1$ ensures the optimum value for the variance.

Quatember's (2009) approach presents in a uniform way a number of techniques. In Quatember (2012) this standardization is extended to the case of multi-stage setup, so that techniques which require more than two stages are included. Among those techniques are the ones of Mangat and Singh (1990), Mangat (1992), Mangat, Singh, and Singh (1993) and Singh, Singh, Mangat, and Tracy (1995).

The approach just described, covers many models, but does not offer any way to handle techniques which allow for more than just the two "Yes" and "No" answers. The approach developed by Chaudhuri et al. (2009) covers techniques which allow for multiple answers. This is as follows.

Denote by L_i the probability that the unit i of the population belongs to the stigmatizing group. To avoid trivialities we assume that L_i can be neither zero nor one.

Let $L_i(R)$ denote the (conditional) probability that unit i of the population belongs to the stigmatizing group, given that his/her response is R. Then

$$J_i(R) = \frac{L_i(R)/L_i}{[1 - L_i(R)]/(1 - L_i)} \tag{7.7}$$

is regarded as the response-specific measure of jeopardy of participant for the particular randomized response technique.

The above measure of jeopardy depends on the specific response R. It is fair that this measure should be communicated to the participants before they agree to participate, because, such a measure quantifies the risk of revealing one's status about the stigmatizing characteristic. However, given that the measure is response-specific, its value for the various possible responses, especially for randomized response techniques with more than two possible responses, will not be easily accessed by the participants. But even in the case of randomization devices with just two possible answers, the numerical value of the above measure is not really of any value to a participating person. Assume, for instance, that in the Warner's (1965) model a participant responds to the question whether he/she belongs to the stigmatizing group with probability 0.44. Then the values for $J(1)$ and $J(0)$ are 0.785 and 1.272, respectively (assuming here that the value $R = 1$ means that the participant responded "Yes" and similarly the value $R = 0$ corresponds to a "No" response). These values can hardly quantify the risk of revealing one's status about the sensitive attribute. In addition, they could be misunderstood. For example, under the impression that a smaller value protects their privacy better, participants presented with the above two values of 0.785 and 1.272 might be tempted to provide a "Yes" response, the same way that they may be tempted to provide a "No" response if they are presented with the values of 1.439 and 0.694 corresponding to $J(1)$ and $J(0)$, respectively, for the case where the parameter of the randomization device is 0.59. It is therefore reasonable to construct a measure which is not response specific

7.2 Measures of Jeopardy

but rather takes into consideration all possible responses. Such a new measure can be regarded as a technical specification of the randomization device and should be made known to the participants before they agree to participate in the survey. Chaudhuri et al. (2009) proposed the following measure:

$$\bar{J}_i = \frac{1}{M} \sum_R J_i(R), \tag{7.8}$$

where M is the number of possible responses of the particular randomized response technique and the summation is taken over all possible responses. This measure takes on a single value. Values close to unity are those that are taken to guarantee the protection of privacy of the i-th participant. We will display the above measure for the following techniques: Warner's (1965) model, Kuk's (1990) procedure, Mangat and Singh's (1990) technique, Christofides' (2003) technique and the Three Sample Item Count Technique. Warner's (1965) and Mangat and Singh's (1990) allow only for two possible responses whereas the remaining techniques allow for more than two.

For Warner's (1965) technique with randomization parameter p the above measure is calculated as follows:

For the i unit of the population, let I_i denote his/her randomized response, i.e., I_i takes one the value 1 if i responds "Yes" and the value 0 if i responds "No." Then,

$$L_i(1) = \frac{L_i P(I_i = 1 \mid y_i = 1)}{L_i P(I_i = 1 \mid y_i = 1) + (1 - L_i) P(I_i = 1 \mid y_i = 0)}$$
$$= \frac{pL_i}{(1-p) + (2p-1)L_i} \tag{7.9}$$

and

$$L_i(0) = \frac{L_i P(I_i = 0 \mid y_i = 1)}{L_i P(I_i = 0 \mid y_i = 1) + (1 - L_i) P(I_i = 0 \mid y_i = 0)}$$
$$= \frac{(1-p)L_i}{p + (1-2p)L_i} \tag{7.10}$$

Using (7.9) and (7.10) in (7.7) we find that

$$J_i(1) = \frac{p}{1-p} \text{ and } J_i(0) = \frac{1-p}{p}.$$

From (7.8) it follows that

$$\bar{J}_i = \frac{J_i(1) + J_i(0)}{2} = \frac{1}{2}\left(\frac{p}{1-p} + \frac{1-p}{p}\right).$$

Observe that with $p \to 0.5$, $\bar{J}_i \to 1$, but of course in such a case the variance of the estimator goes to infinity.

For Kuk's (1990) model, $\bar{J}_i$ can be calculated in a similar manner. Recall first that under this technique, participant i is presented with two boxes containing identical cards of red and white color. Assume that in each box we have sufficiently large numbers of cards and the proportion of red cards in the two boxes are p_1 and p_2, respectively. A person sampled is requested to use the first box, if he/she has the stigmatizing characteristic and the second box if not. The use of the box consists of k independent draws of cards with replacement and the participant is to report to the interviewer the number of times a red card is drawn, denoted by f_i. Then we can calculate the following quantities:

$$L_i(f_i) = \frac{L_i\left[p_1^{f_i}(1-p_1)^{k-f_i}\right]}{p_2^{f_i}(1-p_2)^{k-f_i} + L_i\left[p_1^{f_i}(1-p_1)^{k-f_i} - p_2^{f_i}(1-p_2)^{k-f_i}\right]}$$

and

$$J_i(f_i) = \frac{p_1^{f_i}(1-p_1)^{k-f_i}}{p_2^{f_i}(1-p_2)^{k-f_i}}.$$

Then,

$$\bar{J}_i = \frac{1}{k+1}\sum_{f_i=0}^{k} J_i(f_i).$$

Observe that, in a similar way to the behavior of the above quantity in Warner's model, $\bar{J}_i \to 1$, as $p_1 \to p_2$, but at the same time the variance of the estimator goes to infinity.

For Mangat and Singh's (1990) device we can calculate the relevant measures of jeopardy. First recall that in this technique a sampled person i is provided with two randomization devices, which must be used in the absence of the interviewer. Using the first randomization device, the sampled person, is instructed with probability T $(0 < T < 1)$ to respond truthfully (with a "Yes" or "No") whether he/she has the stigmatizing characteristic and with probability $1 - T$ to use the second randomization device which is exactly the same as in Warner's technique with parameter p. Then

$$L_i(1) = \frac{L_i[T + (1-T)p]}{(1-T)(1-p) + L_i[T + (1-T)(2p-1)]} = \frac{L_i(\alpha + \beta)}{\beta + L_i\alpha},$$

$$L_i(0) = \frac{L_i(1-T)(1-p)}{T + p(1-T) + L_i[T + (1-T)(2p-1)]} = \frac{L_i\beta}{\alpha + \beta - L_i\alpha},$$

7.2 Measures of Jeopardy

where $\alpha = T + (1-T)(2p-1)$ and $\beta = (1-T)(1-p)$. In addition,

$$J_i(1) = \frac{\alpha + \beta}{\beta} \text{ and } J_i(0) = \frac{\beta}{\alpha + \beta}.$$

Then

$$\bar{J}_i = \frac{1}{2}[J_i(0) + J_i(1)] = \frac{1}{2}\left(\frac{\beta}{\alpha + \beta} + \frac{\alpha + \beta}{\beta}\right).$$

Observe that $\bar{J}_i \to 1$, as $\alpha \to 0$. However, from Sect. 4.4.3,

$$V_i = (1-T)(1-p)\left[T + p(1-T)\right] = \frac{\beta(1-\beta)}{\alpha^2}$$

which means that $V_i \to \infty$, as $\alpha \to 0$.

For the Christofides (2003) device, recall that a sample person is required to generate one of the numbers $1, \ldots, M$ using a random mechanism which produces these numbers with respective probabilities $p_1, \ldots, p_M$, with $0 < p_j < 1$, $j = 1, \ldots, M$ and $\sum_{j=1}^{M} p_j = 1$. Then he/she is to report the number generated, say k, if he/she does not belong to the sensitive group, or the number $M+1-k$ otherwise. We can easily calculate the quantities,

$$L_i(k) = \frac{L_i p_{M+1-k}}{p_k + L_i(p_{M+1-k} - p_k)}, \quad k = 1, \ldots, M,$$

and

$$J_i(k) = \frac{p_{M+1-k}}{p_k}, \quad k = 1, \ldots, M.$$

Therefore,

$$\bar{J}_i = \frac{1}{M}\sum_{k=1}^{M}\left(\frac{p_{M+1-k}}{p_k}\right).$$

It can be easily verified that as $p_k \to (1/M)$ for $k = 1, \ldots, M$, then $\bar{J}_i \to 1$, while $V_i \to \infty$, verifying once more that the protection of privacy and efficiency move to opposite directions.

For the Three Sample Item Count Technique as described in Sect. 6.2.2, let X_i be the number reported by the i-th individual of the first sample. Then $L_i(k) = P(y_i = 1|X_i = k)$ is defined for $k = 0, 1, \ldots, G+1$. Clearly, $L_i(0) = 0$ and consequently, $J_i(0) = 0$. Observe that for $k = 1, \ldots, G$,

$$P(X_i = k \mid y_i = 1) = p_{k-1},$$

and
$$P(X_i = k \mid y_i = 0) = p_k(1 - \theta_F) + p_{k-1}\theta_F.$$

Furthermore, $P(X_i = G+1 \mid y_i = 1) = p_G$ and $P(X_i = G+1 \mid y_i = 0) = \theta_F p_G$. Then for $k = 1, \ldots, G$

$$L_i(k) = \frac{L_i P(X_i = k \mid y_i = 1)}{L_i P(X_i = k \mid y_i = 1) + (1 - L_i) P(X_i = k \mid y_i = 0)}$$

$$= \frac{L_i p_{k-1}}{L_i p_{k-1} + (1 - L_i)[p_k(1 - \theta_F) + p_{k-1}\theta_F]}.$$

Therefore,

$$J_i(k) = \frac{L_i(k)(1 - L_i)}{[1 - L_i(k)] L_i} = \frac{p_{k-1}}{p_k(1 - \theta_F) + p_{k-1}\theta_F}, \quad k = 1, \ldots, G.$$

Finally,

$$L_i(G+1) = \frac{L_i p_G}{L_i p_G + (1 - L_i)\theta_F p_G} = \frac{L_i}{L_i + (1 - L_i)\theta_F}$$

and

$$J_i(G+1) = \frac{L_i(G+1)(1 - L_i)}{[1 - L_i(G+1)] L_i} = \frac{1}{\theta_F}.$$

The measure of jeopardy therefore takes the form

$$\bar{J}_i = \frac{1}{G+1}\left[\sum_{k=1}^{G} \frac{p_{k-1}}{p_k(1 - \theta_F) + p_{k-1}\theta_F} + \frac{1}{\theta_F}\right].$$

Based on the above, it is clear that with $\theta_F \to 1$ or with $(p_{k-1}/p_k) \to 1$, $J_i(k) \to 1$ for $k = 1, \ldots, G$, while as $\theta_F \to 0$, $J_i(G+1) \to \infty$ as expected.

Considering the same quantities but for a respondent from the second sample we have the following:

$$L_i(0) = 0 \text{ and } J_i(0) = 0$$

and for $k = 1, \ldots, G$,

$$P(X_i = k \mid y_i = 1) = p_{k-1},$$

7.2 Measures of Jeopardy

and

$$P(X_i = k \mid y_i = 0) = p_k \theta_F + p_{k-1}(1 - \theta_F).$$

In addition,

$$P(X_i = G + 1 \mid y_i = 1) = p_G$$

and

$$P(X_i = G + 1 \mid y_i = 0) = p_G(1 - \theta_F).$$

Then, for $k = 1, \ldots, G$

$$L_i(k) = \frac{L_i P(X_i = k \mid y_i = 1)}{L_i P(X_i = k \mid y_i = 1) + (1 - L_i) P(X_i = k \mid y_i = 0)}$$

$$= \frac{L_i p_{k-1}}{L_i p_{k-1} + (1 - L_i)[p_k \theta_F + p_{k-1}(1 - \theta_F)]}.$$

Consequently,

$$J_i(k) = \frac{L_i(k)(1 - L_i)}{[1 - L_i(k)] L_i} = \frac{p_{k-1}}{p_k \theta_F + p_{k-1}(1 - \theta_F)}, \quad k = 1, \ldots, G.$$

Furthermore,

$$L_i(G + 1) = \frac{L_i p_G}{L_i p_G + (1 - L_i)(1 - \theta_F) p_G} = \frac{L_i}{L_i + (1 - L_i)(1 - \theta_F)}$$

which gives

$$J_i(G + 1) = \frac{L_i(G + 1)(1 - L_i)}{[1 - L_i(G + 1)] L_i} = \frac{1}{1 - \theta_F}.$$

Thus,

$$\bar{J}_i = \frac{1}{G + 1} \left[\sum_{k=1}^{G} \frac{p_{k-1}}{p_k \theta_F + p_{k-1}(1 - \theta_F)} + \frac{1}{1 - \theta_F} \right].$$

Obviously, we find that as $\theta_F \to 0$ or as $\frac{p_{k-1}}{p_k} \to 1$, $J_i(k) \to 1$ for $k = 1, \ldots, G$, while as $\theta_F \to 1$, $J_i(G + 1) \to \infty$ as expected.

Given that this measure is a technical characteristic of the randomization device, i.e., it solely depends on the probabilities with which one provides each one of the possible answers, one may wonder why not choose these probabilities so that this measure is as small as possible. The answer lies on the fact that the variance of the unbiased estimator generated moves to the opposite direction. This means that the smaller the value of $\bar{J}_i$, the greater the variance of the estimator and vice versa. So, a common sense mandates that the parameters of the randomization device should be so chosen that both the measure of jeopardy and the variance of the estimator are maintained at acceptable levels.

The necessity to adopt a measure such as the one given by (7.8) arises also from the fact that most measures of privacy protection have been devised to accommodate randomized response techniques in which participants provide just a "Yes" or a "No" answer. However, as already mentioned, some techniques allow for multiple responses, for example Kuk (1990) and Christofides (2003).

Nayak and Adeshiyan (2009) adopt the following approach for techniques allowing for multiple responses.

Let Y be the indicator of the stigmatizing characteristic, i.e., $Y = 1$ if the respondent belongs to the sensitive group and $Y = 0$, if not. Denote by Z the response variable and the k different responses by $c_1, \ldots, c_k$. Finally denote the quantities $P(Z = c_i | Y = 1)$ and $P(Z = c_i | Y = 0)$ by α_i and β_i, respectively, for $i = 1, \ldots, k$. The quantity

$$R\left(\underline{\alpha}, \underline{\beta}\right) = \max\left\{\frac{\alpha_1}{\beta_1}, \ldots, \frac{\alpha_k}{\beta_k}\right\}$$

is taken as a measure of the degree of privacy.

Although there exist measures which deal with techniques with multiple responses, for example, the one by Nayak and Adeshiyan (2009) just presented, by construction, those measures do not really do justice to techniques with multiple responses. See, for example, the arguments in Christofides (2010).

One may wonder however, whether the participants are in a position to appreciate the value of the above measure of jeopardy (or any measure for that matter). What is important from the participants' point of view is not really the measure of jeopardy but their perception as to whether their privacy is protected by the randomized response technique, or by the indirect questioning technique in general. This is an issue discussed in Sect. 7.4.

7.3 Protection of Privacy in Case of Quantitative Sensitive Characteristics

Very little has been done on the issue of privacy protection in case of quantitative sensitive characteristics. Only very recently, Bose (2013) has given a randomized response device exclusively for a discrete real-valued random variable tied to a simple random sample drawn with replacement from the population. We present very briefly the main ideas of Bose (2013).

7.3 Protection of Privacy in Case of Quantitative Sensitive Characteristics

Let X denote the stigmatizing variable of interest and assume that X can take only the (known) values $x_1, \ldots, x_m$, with m a finite integer. Further assume that

$$P(X = x_k) = \theta_k,$$

where $\theta_k \geq 0$ for all $k = 1, \ldots, m$ and $\sum_{k=1}^{m} \theta_k = 1$. Obviously, the mean μ and variance σ^2 of the random variable X are given by

$$\mu = \sum_{k=1}^{m} \theta_k x_k, \quad \sigma^2 = \sum_{k=1}^{m} \theta_k (x_k - \mu)^2.$$

For the purpose of estimating μ, a simple random sample of size n is drawn with replacement from the population. Each participant is provided with a box containing cards of $m + 1$ types. He/she is to draw one card a follow the instruction of the card. The instruction on the kth type card says "Report x_k as your response," for $k = 1, \ldots, m$ while the $(m + 1)$-st type says "Report your true value." The box contains a large number cards with the following composition: Mp of the cards are of the $(m + 1)$-st type and $M(1 - p)/m$ are cards of each of the types k, with M a positive integer and $0 < p < 1$, assuming of course that Mp and $M(1 - p)/m$ are positive integers.

Assuming that R denotes the response provided by a participant, it is easy to verify that

$$P(R = x_k \mid X = x_j) = \frac{1-p}{m}, \text{ for } k = 1, \ldots, m, \; j = 1, \ldots, m, \; k \neq j$$

and

$$P(R = x_j \mid X = x_j) = p + \frac{1-p}{m}, \text{ for } j = 1, \ldots, m.$$

Let w_k be the sample proportion of people reporting x_k as their response and let $\bar{x}$ the sample average of $x_1, \ldots, x_m$. Then Bose (2013) shows that

$$\widehat{\theta_k} = \frac{1}{p}\left(w_k - \frac{1-p}{m}\right)$$

is an unbiased estimator of θ_k for $k = 1, \ldots, m$ and that

$$\hat{\mu} = \frac{1}{p} \sum_{k=1}^{m} w_k x_k - \frac{1-p}{p} \bar{x}$$

is an unbiased estimator of μ with variance given by

$$V(\hat{\mu}) = \frac{1}{np^2}\left[p\sigma^2 + \frac{1-p}{m}\sum_{k=1}^{m}(x_k-\bar{x})^2 + p(p-1)(\mu-\bar{x})^2\right].$$

As a measure of privacy protection, Bose (2013) proposes the following

$$\alpha = \max_{1 \leq k, j \leq m} |P(X = x_k \mid R = x_j) - P(X = x_k)|.$$

The idea behind this measure is that a randomization device with a value of $\alpha = c$ guarantees that the discrepancies between the true and revealing probabilities will be at most c. Bose (2013) shows that if the designer of the survey wants to have α to be at most ξ where $0 < \xi < 1$, then a necessary and sufficient condition is that

$$p \leq \left(1 + \frac{m}{\xi}\left(\frac{1-\xi}{2}\right)^2\right)^{-1}.$$

The above condition is based on the assumption that all values $x_1, \ldots, x_m$ are stigmatizing. Bose (2013) provides a similar result in case where some of the values of the x_k's are not stigmatizing.

The setup in Bose (2013) assumes selection of a simple random sample drawn with replacement from the population about which we have our usual reservation because we are propagating the view that no randomized response technique needs to be tied to any specific sampling scheme, so long as it ensures positive inclusion probabilities for every unit as well as for every pair of distinct units.

In what follows in this section, for two randomized response devices which are common in the literature for estimation of quantitative sensitive characteristics, we discuss the issue of protection of privacy.

Let as usual y_i denote the fixed but unknown value of the stigmatizing real variable y on a person labeled i in a finite survey population $U = (1, \ldots, N)$. The objective is to estimate the total $Y = \sum_{i=1}^{N} y_i$ on obtaining a probability sample s with probability $p(s)$ and eliciting randomized responses as z_i's from respective sampled persons i in s.

7.3.1 Randomized Device I

The investigator approaches a sampled person i in U with a box containing T cards marked $a_1, \ldots, a_j, \ldots, a_T$ with

$$\frac{1}{T}\sum_{i=1}^{T} a_i = \mu_a \neq 0 \text{ and } \frac{1}{T}\sum_{i=1}^{T}(a_i - \mu_a)^2 = \sigma_a^2$$

and a second box containing M cards marked $b_1, \ldots, b_k, \ldots, b_M$ with

7.3 Protection of Privacy in Case of Quantitative Sensitive Characteristics

$$\frac{1}{M}\sum_{k=1}^{M} b_k = \mu_b \text{ and } \frac{1}{M}\sum_{k=1}^{M} (b_k - \mu_b)^2 = \sigma_b^2.$$

The respondent, on request draws one card from the first box marked as a_j, say, and independently draws one card from the second box marked as b_k, say. Without disclosing these two values to the investigator, he/she gives out as his/her randomized response as

$$z_i = a_j y_i + b_k, \quad j = 1, \ldots, T, \quad k = 1, \ldots, M.$$

Recall from Sect. 5.2.1, that

$$E_R(z_i) = y_i \mu_a + \mu_b$$

and

$$V_R(z_i) = y_i^2 \sigma_a^2 + \sigma_b^2.$$

Hence, $r_i = \mu_a^{-1}(z_i - \mu_b)$ unbiased estimates y_i with variance given by

$$V_i = V_R(r_i) = \frac{V_R(z_i)}{\mu_a^2} = y_i^2 \frac{\sigma_a^2}{\mu_a^2} + \frac{\sigma_b^2}{\mu_b^2}.$$

More importantly, each of the above possible values for z_i, for any unknown y_i is assumed with probability $1/(TM)$ for $j = 1, \ldots, T$ and $k = 1, \ldots, M$.

In order to assess how this randomized response device may protect the privacy of a respondent i giving out the randomized response as z_i let us postulate the prior probability $L(y_i) = L_i$ for the value of y_i. We may note that the posterior probability $L(y_i \mid z_i)$ of y_i given the randomized response z_i by means of Bayes theorem turns out to be

$$L(y_i \mid z_i) = \frac{L_i P(z_i \mid y_i)}{P(z_i)}$$
$$= \frac{L_i (1/(TM))}{(1/(TM))}$$
$$= L_i$$

for every i in U, where $P(z_i \mid y_i)$ stands for the conditional probability that respondent i gives z_i as his/her randomized response given that the value of the true characteristic is y_i and $P(z_i)$ denotes the probability that respondent i gives z_i as his/her randomized response.

So the respondent's privacy is protected well for every T and every M. But this is counter-intuitive because if $T = 1$ and $M = 1$, then given z_i, the value of y_i with probability one is revealed as

$$y_i = \frac{z_i - b_1}{a_i}, \quad \forall i \in U.$$

But if $T > 1$ and $M > 1$, even if say $T = 2$ and $M = 2$, one may at most guess the true value of y_i with probability 0.25. So, we may safely conclude that the randomized response device I protects well the privacy of a respondent.

7.3.2 Randomized Response Device II

The investigator requests a sampled person i to draw randomly one card from a box containing a number of cards, a proportion C ($0 < C < 1$) of them marked "true" and others marked $x_1, \ldots, x_j, \ldots, x_M$ with relative frequencies $q_1, \ldots, q_j, \ldots, q_M$ such that $\sum_{j=1}^{M} q_j = 1 - C$. Then a secretly elicited randomized response is

$$z_i = \begin{cases} y_i & \text{if a "true" marked card is drawn} \\ x_j & \text{if an } x_j \text{ marked card is drawn.} \end{cases}$$

Then

$$E_R(z_i) = Cy_i + \sum_{j=1}^{M} q_j x_j,$$

and from Sect. 5.2.2 we conclude that the quantity

$$r_i = \frac{1}{C}\left(z_i - \sum_{j=1}^{M} q_j x_j\right)$$

unbiasedly estimates y_i, for $i \in U$. Also,

$$V_R(z_i) = Cy_i^2 + \sum_{j=1}^{M} q_j x_j^2 - \left(Cy_i + \sum_{j=1}^{M} q_j x_j\right)^2$$

and hence

$$V_i = V_R(r_i) = \frac{1}{C^2} V_R(z_i) = \alpha y_i^2 + \beta y_i + \nu$$

with α, β, ν known. Correspondingly,

$$v_i = \frac{\alpha r_i^2 + \beta r_i + \nu}{1 + \alpha}$$

has $E_R(v_i) = V_i$ for $i \in U$.

A respondent is given to know all the values C, x_j and q_j for $j = 1, \ldots, M$ and so may assess the price of his/her revelation of the values of z_i for each i in U. To judge such a price, let us consider the Bayes posterior probability which is the conditional probability $L(y_i \mid z_i)$ of giving out the value when a value z_i is given corresponding to a postulated prior probability $L(y_i) = L_i$ that one may hit upon. Bayes theorem gives

$$L(y_i \mid z_i) = \frac{L(y_i) C}{L(y_i) C + (1 - L(y_i)) \sum_{j=1}^{M} q_j}$$

$$= \frac{CL_i}{CL_i + (1 - C)(1 - L_i)}$$

$$= \frac{CL_i}{L_i(2C - 1) + (1 - C)}$$

$$= \frac{L_i}{L_i \left(2 - \frac{1}{C}\right) + \left(\frac{1}{C} - 1\right)}.$$

The respondent may feel protected if $L(y_i \mid z_i)$ is close to L_i. So a value of C taken as 0.5 will give him/her the most coveted protection a is intuitively clear, because in this case $L(y_i \mid z_i)$ equals L_i, i.e., given out the response as z_i, the posterior and the prior coincide. As a consequence, when $C = 0.5$ the value of $\sum_{j=1}^{M} q_j$ is equal to 0.5 as well. From this however, no rational conclusion seems possible about the magnitude of $V_R(z_i)$ or $V_R(r_i)$.

7.4 Perceived Protection of Privacy

The main purpose of randomized response and other indirect questioning techniques is to increase participation, reduce nonresponse, and reduce untruthful responses in surveys dealing with stigmatizing characteristics. However, problems have been reported in applying the indirect response methodology which may jeopardize the validity of the results. In some cases, the problems are attributed to the design of questionnaires such as in the case reported by Tsuchiya and Hirai (2010). In most cases however, those problems are related to the perceived risk of disclosure. We refer to the following examples:

Boeije and Lensvelt-Mulders (2002) on page 34 report that "Giving forced answers to a question, in particular when they should be negative, was felt to be dishonest and unpleasant. Individuals who had nothing to hide and who reported all their activities to the Department of Social Services felt afraid that an affirmative answer would have implications. In their eyes even a forced "yes" on one of the questions could harm them; The only way to be completely safe, in their view, is to say "no" in spite of the instructions."

van der Heijden, van Gils, Bouts, and Hox (2000) on page 526 state that "The results are not comforting. Although the RR approach performs much better than more traditional approaches, the percentage of respondents admitting to fraud is far less than 100 percent." The reader should have in mind that the study the authors refer to is a study in which all participants had committed fraud and therefore it is clear that participants either did not follow the rules or did not provide truthful responses.

Coutts and Jann (2011) on page 184 state that "The often negative prevalence estimates obtained with the various versions of RRT indicate that noncompliance with RRT instructions was frequent in our study. Similar results have been reported in other studies, especially those in which a forced-choice method directs respondents to provide an automatic yes answer."

Krebs et al. (2011) on page 231 write that "It should be encouraging, however, to researchers in the field of sexual assault that when victims are given both a direct and an indirect opportunity to report experiencing sexual assault, they are not significantly more likely to do so under the indirect method. There are several reasonable interpretations of our findings. First it may be that the logic underlying the indirect questioning technique is flawed and that respondents are not any more comfortable or likely to report experiencing sexual assault victimization under this approach."

Hubbard, Casper, and Lessler (1989) study the reaction of participants to indirect questioning. They say characteristically on page 547 that "Respondents' reactions to the indirect questioning techniques were mixed. Generally randomized response was not well received. All respondents saw the technique as highly obtrusive and potentially disruptive. While respondents generally understood how to answer item count questions, several respondents commented in oral debriefings that they failed to see the technique as a privacy protection, despite explicit instructions aimed at emphasizing that fact."

In the previous section we discussed the measures of jeopardy from the mathematical point of view. Comparisons between various randomized response techniques are based on those measures and on efficiency matters. Usually, authors compare the protection of privacy offered by two different techniques which have the same efficiency, or compare the efficiency of two techniques which offer the same protection of privacy. Those measures are mathematical objects which (unfortunately) are not easily understood by participants. We state here the opinion expressed by Nathan and Sirken (1988) on page 174 of their manuscript. "Although these measures relate to the protection of the individual, they do so, primarily, from the point of view of the data collecting agency, rather than that of the respondent. Thus, as pointed out by Leysieffer and Warner (1976), they could be considered as relating to the case where data have already been collected by direct questioning and randomization is carried out a-posteriori to protect privacy."

From a practical point of view, one may pose the following question: When is a randomized response (or an indirect questioning) technique considered to be successful? Is it when the risk of disclosure is very low, but perhaps the perceived risk of disclosure is very high and people refuse to participate or is it when

7.4 Perceived Protection of Privacy

people are willing to participate because they believe that their privacy is protected regardless of what the risk of disclosure is?

Common sense mandates that the perceived protection of privacy is crucial in deciding to participate in a survey dealing with sensitive issues. In fact it is gaining ground the opinion that the perception of privacy protection should also be considered when the protection of privacy offered by various indirect questioning techniques is examined. Quatember (2012), for example, implicitly recognizes that certain designs, by construction, may increase the respondents' perceived privacy protection. Furthermore, there is empirical (and scientific) evidence that the perception of risk is very important. Here are some examples:

Lensvelt-Mulders, Hox, and van der Heijden (2005) on page 263 state that "An extra advantage of using a forced response method is that the perceived protection of the respondents can be manipulated. It is a well-known fact that people have incorrect intuitions about the calculation of probabilities. This flaw can be used to the advantage of researchers, by making the subjective privacy protection larger than the true statistical privacy protection."

Couper, Singer, Conrad, and Groves (2008) inform us on pages 256, 271, and 273 that "In an experiment embedded in a monthly telephone survey, Singer (2003) showed that subjective perceptions of disclosure risk, and perceptions of harm from the disclosure of identified information, are highly correlated with expressed willingness to participate in surveys. Nor did the confidentiality assurance significantly affect willingness to participate; in fact, the direction of the coefficient was consistently negative, suggesting that in the circumstances of the present experiment, an assurance of confidentiality may actually have reduced willingness to participate. In the present experiment, as in earlier research, it is respondents' perceptions—their concerns about confidentiality or privacy, their estimations of how likely it is that others will gain access to information about them, and their perceptions of how harmful that would be—that are significantly correlated with willingness to participate in the research. We speculate that what reduces willingness to participate in a survey is not the actual risk of disclosure, but the perceived risk (probability) of anticipated harm from disclosure."

Bockenholt, Barlas, and van der Heijden (2009) stress the necessity to design experiments to see the reaction of participants to randomized response techniques offering different levels of privacy protection. They say on page 390 of their manuscript that "It therefore seems promising to conduct experimental studies that investigate the degree to which respondents distinguish and react positively to the different levels of privacy protection offered by these RR methods."

If the perceived risk of disclosure is important, then how do we measure it? Which techniques do increase the so-called perceived level of the protection of privacy? It is reasonable to assume that for psychological reasons, techniques allowing for multiple responses, for example, Kuk's model, provide a feeling of protection to participants more than say, Warner's technique which mandates for only two possible responses? In addition, we can always use survey methodology (or in some cases qualitative studies) to measure the attitude of participants to two different indirect questioning techniques, but is it possible to do it in order to compare multiple techniques? Can we develop the mathematical methodology so that for each technique we have a single index which measures the perceived protection of privacy? Given that the concept of perception is highly subjective, perhaps we will also need the involvement of scientists from other disciplines. The social sciences in general and cognitive sciences in particular may be crucial in accomplishing such a task.

References

Bockenholt, U., Barlas, S., van der Heijden, P.G.M. (2009). Do randomized response designs eliminate response biases? An empirical study of non compliance behavior. *Journal of Applied Economics, 24*, 377–392.

Boeije, H., & Lensvelt-Mulders, G. (2002). Honest by chance: a qualitative interview study to clarify respondents' (non-) compliance with computer assisted randomized response. *Bulletin Methodologie Sociologique, 75*, 24–39.

Bose, M. (2013). Respondent privacy and estimation efficiency in randomized response surveys for disctrete-valued sensitive variables. arXiv:1303.5172v1.

Chaudhuri, A., Christofides, T.C., Saha, A. (2009). Protection of privacy in efficient application of randomized response techniques. *Statistical Methods and Applications, 18*, 389–418.

Chaudhuri, A., & Saha, A. (2004). Utilizing covariates by logistic regression modeling in improved estimation of population proportions bearing stigmatizing features through randomized responses in complex surveys. *Journal of the Indian Society of Agricultural Statistics, 58*, 190–211.

Christofides, T.C. (2003). A generalized randomized response technique. *Metrika, 57*, 195–200.

Christofides, T.C. (2010). Comments on a method of comparison of randomized response techniques. *Journal of Statistical Planning and Inference, 140*, 574–575.

Couper, M.P., Singer, E., Conrad, F.G., Groves, R.M. (2008). Risk of disclosure, perceptions of risk, and concerns about privacy and confidentiality as factors in survey participation. *Journal of Official Statistics, 24*, 255–275.

Coutts, E., & Jann, B. (2011). Sensitive questions in online surveys: experimental results for the randomized response technique (RRT) and the unmatched count technique (UCT). *Sociological Methods & Research, 40*, 169–193.

Greenberg, B.G., Abul-Ela, A.-L.A., Simmons, W.R., Horvitz, D.G. (1969). The unrelated question RR model: theoretical framework. *Journal of the American Statistical Association, 64*, 520–539.

Guerriero, M., & Sandri, M.F. (2007). A note on the comparison of some randomized response procedures. *Journal of Statistical Planning and Inference, 137*, 2184–2190.

Hong, Z., Yan, Z., Wei, L. (2010). A note of proposed privacy measures in randomized response models. *Advances in Intelligent and Soft Computing, 77*, 635–642.

Hubbard, M.L., Casper, R.A., Lessler, J.T. (1989). Respondent reactions to item count lists and randomized response. In *Proceedings of the Survey Research Section of the American Statistical Association*, ASA, 544–548.

Krebs, C.P., Lindquist, C.H., Warner, T.D., Fisher, B.S., Martin, S.L., Childers, J.M. (2011). Comparing sexual assault prevalence estimates obtained with direct and indirect questioning techniques. *Violence Against Women, 17*, 219–235.

Kuk, A.Y.C. (1990). Asking sensitive questions indirectly. *Biometrika, 77*, 436–438.

Lanke, J. (1976). On the degree of protection in randomized interviews. *International Statistical Review, 44*, 197–203.

Lensvelt-Mulders, G.J.L.M., Hox, J.J., van der Heijden, P.G.M. (2005). How to improve the efficiency of randomized response designs. *Quality and Quantity, 39*, 253–265.

References

Leysieffer, F.W., & Warner, S.L. (1976). Respondent jeopardy and optimal designs in randomized response models. *Journal of the American Statistical Association, 71*, 649–656.

Ljungqvist, L. (1993). A unified approach to measures of privacy in randomized response models: a utilitarian perspective. *Journal of the American Statistical Association, 88*, 97–103.

Mangat, N.S. (1992). Two stage randomized response sampling procedure using unrelated question. *Journal of the Indian Society of Agricultural Statistics, 44*, 82–87.

Mangat, N.S., Singh, S., Singh, R. (1993). On the use of modified randomization device in randomized response inquires. *Metron, 51*, 211–216.

Mangat, N.S., Singh, R. (1990). An alternative randomized response procedure. *Biometrika, 77*, 439–442.

Nathan, G., Sirken, M.G. (1988). Cognitive aspects of randomized response. In *Proceedings of the Survey Research Section of the American Statistical Association* (pp. 173–178). Washington DC: American Statistical Association.

Nayak, T.K. (1994). On randomized response surveys for estimating a proportion. *Communications in Statistics-Theory and Methods, 23*, 3303–3321.

Nayak, T.K., & Adeshiyan, S.A. (2009). A unified framework for analysis and comparison of randomized response surveys of binary characteristics. *Journal of Statistical Planning and Inference, 139*, 2757–2766.

Quatember, A. (2009). A standardization of randomized response strategies. *Survey Methodology, 35*, 143–152.

Quatember, A. (2012). An extension of the standardized randomized response technique to a multi-stage setup. *Statistical Methods and Applications, 21*, 475–484.

Singer, E. (2003). Exploring the meaning of consent: participation in research and beliefs about risks and benefits. *Journal of Official Statistics, 19*, 273–285.

Singh, R., Singh, S., Mangat, N.S., Tracy, D.S. (1995). An improved two stage randomized response strategy. *Statistical Papers, 36*, 265–271.

Tsuchiya, T., & Hirai, Y. (2010). Elaborate item count questioning: why do people underreport in item count responses? *Survey Research Methods, 4*, 139–149.

van der Heijden, P.G.M., van Gils, G., Bouts, J., Hox, J. (2000). A comparison of randomized response, Computer assisted Self Interview, and Face to Face Direct Questioning; eliciting sensitive information in the context of welfare and unemployment benefit. *Sociological Methods and Research, 28*, 505–537.

Warner, S.L. (1965). Randomized response: a survey technique for eliminating evasive answer bias. *Journal of the American Statistical Association, 60*, 63–69.

Index

Abernathy, J.R., 5
Abul-Ela, A.-L.A., 3, 32, 73, 91, 153, 154
Academic dishonesty, 2, 142, 143
Adaptive sample, 132
Additive scrambling, 105
Adeshiyan, S.A., 152, 162
Adhikary, A.K., 76
Alhassan, A.W., 90
An, S.-W., 88
Anti-Semitism, 5
Arnab, R., 5, 91, 109–112
Asghari, F., 4, 143

Bagusat, C., 3
Barabesi, L., 77, 84, 85, 88
Bar-Lev, S.K., 5, 88
Barlas, S., 169
Basu, D., 11, 88
Bayes estimator, 86–88, 90
Bayes theorem, 165
Belser, P., 132
Beta distribution, 86
Bias, 11
Biemer, P., 126
Black, S., 4
Block total response, 117
Bobovitch, E., 5, 88
Bockenholt, U., 69, 169
Boeije, H., 167
Boruch, R.F., 3, 33, 46
Bose, M., 131, 132, 162–164
Boukai, B., 5, 88
Bourke, P.D., 84
Bouts, J., 3, 168
Bouza, C.N., 5
Brown, G., 126

Casper, R.A., 168
Chang, H.-J., 90
Chaudhuri, A., 5, 12, 16, 17, 19, 21, 23–25, 33, 34, 46, 53, 55, 58, 61, 62, 65, 73, 76, 88, 91, 95, 100, 102, 103, 117, 120, 129, 131, 132, 143, 146, 152, 153, 156, 157
Chebyshev's inequality, 11
Childers, J.M., 126, 168
Chow, L.P., 57
Christofides' device, 49
Christofides, T.C., 22, 25, 33, 49, 51, 52, 77, 78, 80, 81, 91, 117, 138, 141, 152, 153, 156, 157, 159, 162
Cisin, I.H., 24, 117
Cochran, W.G., 39, 48
Coefficient of variation, 17, 19, 36, 40, 52, 62
Computer assisted self interviewing, 3
Confidence coefficient, 11
Confidence interval, 11
Conrad, F.G., 169
Couper, M.P., 169
Coutts, E., 4, 126, 143, 168
Crossed model, 81, 83
Crosswise model, 4
Covariance operator, 30, 110
Cross-wise non randomized response model, 136
Cruyff, M.J.L.F., 69

Dalenius, T., 53, 54, 56
Danailova-Trainor, G., 132
Device free technique, 25
Devore, J.L., 88
Diana, G., 5
Dietz, P., 3, 4

Dihidar, K., 132
Dihidar, S., 76
Direct survey, 3, 26, 34, 36, 40
Doping, 4
Droitcour, J.A., 25, 116, 132–134

Eichhorn, B.H., 103, 104, 129
Edwards-Jones, G., 4, 132
Eichhorn and Hayre scrambling procedure, 103
Elam, M.E., 91
Emrich, E., 4
Ericson, W.A., 88
Esponda, F., 22, 26, 144, 146, 147
Euro-Justis Survey, 4
Expectation operator, 10, 17, 30, 70, 74, 110, 120, 140

Face-to-face interviewing, 3
Federer, W.F., 117
Finite population, 9, 11, 29, 100, 109
Fisher, B.S., 126, 168
Fligner, M.A., 88
Forced response technique, 3, 33, 46
Fotouhi, A., 4, 143
Fox, J.A., 46
Franceschi, S., 77, 84, 85
Franke, G.A., 3, 4
Franklin, L.A., 84, 86–88

Gaussian negative survey, 146
Gavin, M., 4
Gelfand, A.E., 88
Geng, Z., 22, 25, 134, 135
Geometric distribution, 69
Ghosh, J.K., 131
Gibbons, J.M., 4, 132
Gibbs sampling, 88
Godambe, V.P., 12, 13, 34
Greenberg, B.G., 3, 5, 32, 73, 91, 153, 154
Grewal, I.S., 69, 70, 77
Group testing, 91
Groves, R.M., 169
Grundy, P.M., 15, 31, 45, 136
Guerrero, V.M., 22, 144, 146, 147
Guerriero, M., 152
Gupta, B., 103, 129
Gupta, S., 91, 103, 105, 129

Hajek's ratio estimator, 13
Hansel, J., 4

Hanuvar, T.V., 12
Harrel, A.V., 24, 117
Hartley, H.O., 39, 48
Hastings, W.K., 88
Hayre, L.S., 103, 104, 129
Hege, V.S., 12
Hejri, M.S., 4, 143
Hirai, Y., 126, 167
Hoffman, I., 3
Homogeneous linear unbiased estimator, 12, 96
Hong, K., 91
Hong, Z., 152
Horvitz, D.G., 3, 5, 12, 32, 73, 91, 153, 154
Horvitz-Thompson estimator, 12, 13, 42, 55, 101, 111, 119, 120, 136, 139
Hox, J., 3, 168, 169
Huang, K.-C., 5, 88, 90, 91, 105, 108, 129
Hubbard, M.L., 168
Hussain, Z., 88, 126

Illegal drug use, 4
Imai, K., 126
Induced abortion, 5, 128
Item count question, 4
Item count technique, 4, 22, 24, 116, 117, 126, 127, 157, 159

Jackson, J., 4
Jan, B., 4
Jann, B., 4, 126, 143, 168
Jerk, J., 143
Jerke, J., 4
Joarder, A.H., 64, 91
John, F.A.V.St., 4, 132
Jones, J.P.G., 4, 132

Kadane, J.B., 87
Karlan, D.S., 4
Kerkvliet, J., 3
Kim, J.-M., 69, 88, 91
Klein, M., 4
Krebs, C.P., 126, 168
Krumpal, I., 4, 143
Kuebler, R.R., 5
Kuha, J., 4
Kuk, A.Y.C., 3, 33, 43, 44, 69, 71, 157, 158, 162, 169
Kuk-Revised technique, 72
Kuk's device, 43, 44
Kulik, L., 146
Kunte, S., 88

Kuo, M.-P., 5
Kutnik, B., 132

Lakshmi, D.V., 90
Lan, C.-H., 5
Land, M., 65–67
Lanke, J., 12, 153
Larson, E.M., 25, 116, 132–134
Lee, C.-S., 77, 81, 83
Lee, G.-S., 69, 91
Lee, H., 91
Lensvelt-Mulders, G., 167, 169
Lessler, J.T., 168
Leysieffer, F.W., 153, 168
Lieb, K., 3, 4
Lindquist, C.H., 126, 168
Linear estimator, 64
Linear unbiased estimator, 13
List experiments, 117
Liu, P.T., 57
Ljungqvist, L., 152

Maddala, G.S., 3
Mahmood, M., 5
Mangat, N.S., 59, 61–64, 88, 91, 156–158
Marcheselli, M., 77, 84, 85, 88
Martin, S.L., 126, 168
Maximum likelihood estimator, 66, 86, 88, 139, 146
Mean square error, 10, 16
Measure of jeopardy, 156, 158, 160, 162, 168
Metropolis, N., 88
Migon, H.S., 87
Miller, J.D., 24, 25, 117, 129
Mood enhancement, 4
Moshagen, M., 77
Mosley, W.H., 57
Mukerjee, R., 33, 46, 53, 58, 95, 103, 146
Multinomial distribution, 118, 119, 124, 145, 146
Multiplicative scrambling, 103, 105
Multi-stage sampling, 34
Musch, J., 77
Myers, R.H., 70

Naeher, A.-F., 4, 143
Nathan, G., 168
Nayak, T.K., 152, 153, 162
Negative binomial distribution, 77
Negative question, 116, 144
Negative questionnaire, 26

Negative survey, 22, 26, 144
Network, 131
Network sampling, 24, 25
Neyman, J., 11
Niess, A.M., 4
Nominative technique, 4, 22, 25, 116, 129, 132
Non randomized response model, 4, 22, 25, 26, 116, 134, 141, 143
Normal distribution, 146
Normed size-measure, 39, 76, 100

Observation unit, 24, 130
O'Hagan, A., 87
Ohichi, S., 90
Optional randomized response, 91, 103, 104

Pal, S., 5, 120
Perceived protection of privacy, 26, 152, 169, 170
Perri, P.F., 5
Personal data protection, 2
Peterson, R.A., 3
Pharmacological cognitive enhancement, 4
Pitsch, W., 4
Pitz, G.F., 87
Plagiarism, 4
Poisson distribution, 65–67, 69
Policello, G.E., 88
Polychotomous attribute, 53
Population mean, 10
Population total, 10, 16
Population variance, 10
Positive inclusion probability, 23, 47, 62, 63, 74, 75, 101
Positive questionnaire, 26
Positive question survey, 26
Posterior probability, 89, 165, 167
Post-stratification, 77
Prior probability, 89, 165
Probability proportional to size, 53
Protection of privacy, 2, 3, 24–26, 36, 117, 129, 151–153, 156, 162, 164, 168

Quatember, A., 152, 153, 155, 156, 169

Racism, 4
Raghavarao, D., 90, 117
Randomization device, 2, 24, 25, 30, 31, 33, 37, 51, 52, 60, 62, 63, 66, 70, 78, 81, 84, 98, 110, 116, 141, 157, 161, 162, 164, 165

Randomized response technique, 2–4, 22, 23, 25, 30, 34, 64, 73, 85, 87, 156, 168
Rao, J.K.N., 39, 48
Rao-Hartley-Cochran estimator, 39, 100
Rao-Hartley-Cochran scheme, 39, 43, 45, 48, 52, 62, 74, 76, 100
Rashidian, A., 4, 143
Ratio estimator, 81
Restrictive adaptive sample, 132
Rosenbluth, A.W., 88
Rosenbluth, M.N., 88

Saha, A., 5, 91, 152, 153, 156, 157
Sampling design, 10–12, 14, 19, 30, 36, 39, 47, 58, 64, 70, 74, 101, 112, 120, 136, 155
Sandri, M.F., 152
Scheers, N.J., 3
Scheuren, F.J., 116, 132–134
Seber, G.A.F., 129, 131
Sedory, S.A., 65–67, 77, 81, 83
Sehra, S., 91, 105
Selection unit, 24, 130
Sen, P.K., 5
Sensitivity level, 88, 104
Sexism, 4
Shabbir, J., 88, 91, 105, 126
Shah, B.V., 32, 73
Shannon's uncertainty measure, 144
Sheuren, F.J., 25
Simon, P., 3, 4
Simmons, W.R., 3, 32, 33, 40, 62, 73, 87, 88, 91, 153, 154
Simmon's device, 61
Simmons-Revised technique, 73
Simple model, 81
Simple random sample without replacement, 36, 39, 53, 62, 74, 111
Simple random sample with replacement, 16, 22, 24, 25, 32–34, 46, 49, 54, 58, 62, 64, 67, 69, 76, 81, 86–88, 119, 162, 164
Singer, E., 169
Singh, J., 88
Singh, R., 59, 61, 62, 88, 156–158
Singh, S., 5, 62, 64–67, 69, 70, 77, 81, 83, 91, 103, 129, 156
Sirken, M.G., 168
Smith, A.F.M., 88
Square error loss function, 87
Standard error, 11, 62
Stratified sample, 69

Striegel, H., 3, 4
Survey population, 9

Tachibana, V.M., 87
Taguri, M., 90
Tamhane, A.C., 77
Tan, M.T., 22, 134, 135
Tang, M.L., 22, 25, 134, 135
Tanin, E., 146
Tebbs, J.M., 88
Teller, A.H., 88
Teller, E., 88
Thompson, D.J., 12
Thompson, S.K., 129, 131
Three card method, 22, 116, 132
Tian, G.-L., 22, 25, 134, 135
Tierney, L., 87
Tracy, D.S., 5, 156
Tracy, P.E., 46
Triangular non randomized response model, 136
Tsuchiya, T., 126, 167
Two-stage procedure, 88

Uhm, D., 69, 91
Ulrich, R., 3, 4
Umesh, U.N., 3
Unbiased estimator, 11
Unequal probability sampling, 24, 53
Uniclustered class of designs, 12
Uniformly minimum variance, 12
Unikrishnan, N.K., 88
Unmatched count technique, 117
Unrelated question model, 3, 40, 62, 153, 154
Urlich, R., 4

van der Heijden, P.G.M., 3, 69, 168, 169
van der Hout, A., 69
van Gils, G., 3, 168
Variance operator, 17, 30, 70, 74, 110, 120, 140
Vitale, R.A., 53, 54, 56

Walpole, R.E., 70
Wang, C.-L., 90
Warde, W.D., 91
Warner, S.L., 1, 2, 22, 23, 31–33, 35, 37, 40, 42, 47, 51, 53, 60, 61, 63, 64, 70, 86–89, 91, 141, 153, 154, 157, 168

Warner, T.D., 126, 168
Warner-Revised technique, 70, 72
Wei, L., 152
Winkler, R.L., 86–88

Xenophobia, 4
Xie, H., 146

Yan, Z., 152
Yates, F., 15, 31, 45, 136
Yates-Grundy estimator, 42
Yu, J.-W., 22, 25, 134, 135
Yum, J., 91

Zendehdel, K., 4, 143
Zinman, J., 4

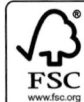

MIX
Papier aus verantwortungsvollen Quellen
Paper from responsible sources
FSC® C105338

If you have any concerns about our products,
you can contact us on
ProductSafety@springernature.com

In case Publisher is established outside the EU,
the EU authorized representative is:
**Springer Nature Customer Service Center GmbH
Europaplatz 3, 69115 Heidelberg, Germany**

Printed by Libri Plureos GmbH
in Hamburg, Germany